The Best
Medicine

Also by Mike Magee, M.D.

The Fifty Most Positive Doctors in America

The Principles of Positive Leadership

Also by Michael D'Antonio

Atomic Harvest

Heaven on Earth

Fall From Grace

The Best Medicine

~

Doctors, Patients, and the Covenant of Caring

Mike Magee, M.D.,
and Michael D'Antonio

St. Martin's Press ✹ New York

THOMAS DUNNE BOOKS.
An imprint of St. Martin's Press.

Book design by Donna Sinisgalli

Library of Congress Cataloging-in-Publication Data

Magee, Mike, M.D.
The best medicine : doctors, patients, and the covenant of caring
/ Mike Magee and Michael D'Antonio.—1st ed.
p.   cm.
ISBN 0-312-24184-4
1. Physician and patient Case studies.   2. Physician and patient
Anecdotes.   I. D'Antonio, Michael.   II. Title.
R727.3.M34   1999
610.69′6—DC21   99-15937
CIP

First Edition: November 1999

1   3   5   7   9   10   8   6   4   2

Dedicated to
the patients and doctors
who opened their lives to us

Contents

Acknowledgments

We thank the individual physicians, general and specialty medical societies, and hospital associations throughout the United States who nominated doctors and patients for interviews. This book would not have been possible without the help of Dilia Santana, Eneida Clarke, and Jo Anne Blakely. Finally, we offer our gratitude to our families for their support and patience with our project.

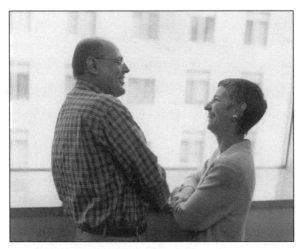

Dr. Jamie Van Roen

The Best
Medicine

Introduction

The patient-physician relationship is the heart of health care. Most of us understand this truth. Think about how much effort we put into finding just the right doctor and how much we value that connection when we make it. Then consider how vital it is to have that relationship when a true crisis arises. The patient-physician relationship may not dominate our lives day by day. But there are moments, for all of us, when nothing is more important. Sometimes a good relationship can even mean the difference between life and death.

The patient-physician relationship has been recognized since Hippocrates and valued through the centuries. It has evolved steadily, yet remained remarkably consistent. Behind closed doors, two individuals—one with a need and the willingness to trust, the other with knowledge and a willingness to respond—seek healing. They form a covenant of caring, a blend of science and humanity that is unique to the needs of one doctor and one patient at one time.

In our time, the traditional view of the positive patient-physician relationship has been challenged, especially by critics of the medical profession, which they see as overly cold and technical. Similarly, managed care and other insurance systems now sometimes come between patients and doctors. We worry about getting access to physicians and having the time to build relationships. This experience can make us feel insecure and even angry.

And it makes it easy to caricature patient-physician interactions as mechanical, or dominated by a kind of paternalism on the physician's part.

If the negative stereotype were true, we might expect people to shy away from the doctor's office. But, in fact, people depend on physicians more than ever. Patients visited doctors more than 730 million times in 1998—2.8 visits for every American man, woman, and child. We know that 75 percent of the population visited a physician this year and that 90 percent did so within the past three years.

The gross numbers tell us that patients still rely on doctors, but they tell us nothing about the quality of their experience. Recently the Pfizer Medical Humanities Initiative conducted a comprehensive nationwide survey of patients and physicians. This work uncovered facts that would confound the critics. Contrary to common belief, patient-physician relationships in America were surprisingly long-term. About 80 percent of patients had relationships with their doctors for an average of seven years. And nearly 30 percent had been with the same doctor for more than ten years.

This is good news because we know that long-term patient-physician relationships are more efficient and effective. The study also showed that the majority of patients and doctors are very satisfied with their relationships. Only about 10 percent expressed dissatisfaction. (This has been confirmed by many other studies and polls, which generally show that concerns about medicine in general are rising, but 80–90 percent of patients rate their own doctors highly.)

Findings on the nature and quality of the relationship are

equally encouraging. According to the study, paternalistic relationships are largely a thing of the past, occurring only in some 10–15 percent of cases. Far more common is a more equal partnership between doctor and patient based on continued scientific advances and active patient education. With the emergence of the patient consumer movement, we have clearly entered an era in which those who deliver care are being guided by those who receive care. Patients are motivating physicians to do more by providing active feedback and raising expectations.

The patient-physician relationship is also less isolated than many of us might assume. Often patients and physicians call on additional caregivers to create a healthcare team. The team may include among others, medical specialists, therapists, hospice care, medical librarians, self-help groups, and even Alzheimer day centers.

How do today's doctors and patients describe their relationships? More than 90 percent of patients and doctors say their relationship is three things. It is compassion. It is understanding, based on active patient education. And it is partnership with shared decision-making.

And who will lead? Who will take charge if one must? Over 90 percent of both doctors and patients say the patient will. Are they ready? An ancient Chinese metaphor suggests they are. In this centuries-old story, patients do not relate to the doctor as a soldier relates to a general. Rather, the patient relates to the doctor as a king to a general, chosen to coordinate the forces against disease.

Dr. Jing-Bao Nie, an expert on Eastern and Western medicine puts it this way, "Wisdom, sincerity, humanity, courage, and strictness constitute the five cardinal virtues of the general. In the Chinese analogy of the physician as General, the good Healer—like the good General—must know the limitations of the art, remain alert to constant changes, cultivate virtues, and fight with humility. Being a General—just as being a physician—is not easy; it requires great wisdom. As the good General sometimes needs to act independent of the opinions of the king, a good king—as a good patient—sometimes accepts the knowledge and the wisdom of the General, acknowledging experience in battle."

The good health of the patient-physician relationship is aided by the fact that the physician's ethical ideals are deliberately high. The American Medical Association states that "medicine is a special kind of human activity—one that cannot be pursued effectively without the traits of humility, honesty, intellectual integrity, compassion, and effacement of excessive self-interest. These traits bind physicians to a moral community dedicated to something other than self-interest."

The tradition of connectedness and intimacy that marks the patient-physician relationship was described by Lewis Thomas as, "The close-up, reassuring, warm touch of the physician, the comfort and concern, the long, leisurely discussions in which everything including the dog can be worked into the conversation . . ."

While today's society is considerably more rushed, patients and physicians continue to favor a relationship-based type of health care. They are seeking balance on many levels in their relationship including decision-making, site of care, methods of communication, and choice of outcome. As one breast cancer survivor told us, "As a patient, there is a delicate balance between how empowered I want to be and how much I want the physician to be in charge. As a cancer survivor, there is no magic 'right' answer about a particular treatment regimen. Even though I want the final decision left to me, it is often confusing and difficult to make the 'right' decision because of different conflicting advice from physicians."

If the patient is challenged, so is the physician who is attempting to balance the cost and quality of care while struggling to consummate a relationship in lesser and lesser amounts of time. Yet, there is evidence that the physician and patient remain remarkably committed to each other and to a common vision of caring that reaffirms Plato's view of the ideal physician. "He learns from the sufferers, and at the same time instructs the invalid to the best of his powers."

This book, *The Best Medicine,* shares the good news revealed in studies, surveys, and our own examination of the state of the patient-physician relationship. Instead of simply reporting the facts, we have allowed doctors and patients to inspire us with their own stories told almost entirely in their own words.

Each of the twenty-five stories is as unique as the characters within them. Where they live, how they feel, who they are, why they believe as they do are different from one to another. But more important than what separates these stories is what connects them. For each is the tale of two human beings, one a patient, the other a doctor, drawn together, in some cases by chance and good luck, and in others by research and good design, to help one another in a moment of human need.

This is also a book about hope, goodness, and possibilities. It displays the finer instincts of our human natures, the ability to survive and even thrive in the face of great challenge and adversity. It suggests that ordinary lives can have extraordinary moments, and that it is not only possible to have an excellent relationship with your doctor, but it is essential.

Most of the doctors featured in this book were nominated by peers who recognized their gift for relating to patients. A few were recommended by patients. Others were discovered by us along the way. All are exemplary in their grasp of medicine as both an art and a science.

Why art and science? Dr. Jing-Bao Nie responds, "Science treats all human beings alike, ignoring dissimilarities to find common features. Medicine must follow science, of course, but it also follows humanities, since a humanistic approach treats every individual as a unique person. This relationship appears totally secular, but there is sacredness in it." In the 1930s, the Boston physician Frances Peabody echoed this sentiment when he said, "There is no more contradiction between the science of medicine and the art of medicine than between the science of aeronautics and the art of flying."

Just as patients are not interchangeable, neither are physicians. Aside from their differing cultures, personalities, and life experiences, they differ in skills and in their willingness to consummate relationships and balance technological and human concerns. All of which is to say that matching a patient to a physician is a highly individualistic and extraordinarily important concern.

But, as you will see in these stories, building such a relationship today is not only valuable, but possible as well. In fact, patients and doctors should settle for nothing less. With these roles come responsibilities. A panel of patients and physicians we convened defined a set of responsibilities that mirror the advice of our patients and physicians.

For the patient:

1. Be truthful: Do not hide facts or exaggerate symptoms. The relationship is based on the free flow of confidentially held and sensitive information. Inaccuracy threatens the patient's health and the relationship. Respect the confidentiality of your communications with your doctor.

2. Give the relationship time: As with all complex human encounters, this relationship needs time to mature and develop. Get to know each other. Be open to a partnership in decision-making.

3. Take responsibility for learning: Mark Twain said, "You might die of a misprint." Your body is complex. Commit to understanding how it functions and how to keep it healthy.

4. Take responsibility for your health: "Know thyself" means more than just knowing what diseases you have and what medications you are on. It also means having a well-defined health philosophy for you and your family. They are partners in this relationship as well.

5. Raise issues of concern: Hidden issues, left unsurfaced, will ultimately compromise even a stellar relationship. If something is bothering you—the doctor's rushing, the staff is rude, the room is cold—whatever, speak up.

For the physician:

1. Act with the highest professional competency: Trust requires a high level of physician competency and the ability to culturally connect and communicate clearly one-on-one.

2. Master the skills of communication: Part of creating a good match is the ability to communicate complex

science in layman's terms and in a neighborly way. Help patients understand and absorb medical developments. Always honor confidentiality.

3. Allow patients to share ideas and help formulate priorities: In an environment where time is a limited commodity, priority setting needs to be collaborative and ideas which are urgent to the patient must be permitted to surface.

4. Acknowledge the fullness of your patient: Wellness and illness are highly individualistic. They must be interpreted within the context of family, job, finances, and mental and spiritual health.

5. Respect your fellow professionals: Patients expect their doctors to work well with each other and with other caregivers. Turf battles are a nightmare for the patient. Open disagreements and rude interprofessional behavior cause patients to question their physicians' credibility and capability.

Not too long ago, we were approached by a third-year medical student who had heard we were collecting stories and wanted to share one of her own. She said that the day before she had been driving in the car with her three-year-old child. She said to the little girl, "You know Mommy wants to be a doctor." Her daughter said, "Uh-huh." She then said, "And you know, Mommy's decided to be the type of doctor who delivers babies." A few minutes later the little girl looked up at her mother and said, "I want to be a doctor, too." The mother responded, "Well, what type of doctor do you want to be?", expecting the girl to want to deliver babies also. The little girl thought for a moment or two, and then looked up at her mother and said, "A nice one!"

What follows are the stories of twenty-five doctors and twenty-five patients, all of them "nice ones."

PART ONE

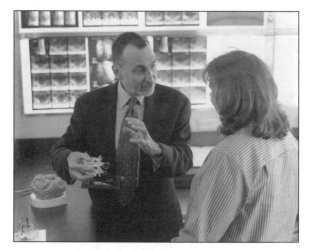

Dr. Stanley Pelofsky

The

Scientists

Dr. Fearless

⌇

Stanley Pelofsky, M.D., 58,
neurosurgeon, Oklahoma City, Oklahoma

Pamela Deen, 46, homemaker, Norman, Oklahoma, and
Natalie Hartman, 18, student, Piedmont, Oklahoma

⌇

PAMELA DEEN, PATIENT

Pamela Deen was facing almost certain death when she met Stanley Pelofsky. Seven years of headaches had finally been diagnosed properly. By then her pituitary tumor was so large she was given only a fifty-fifty chance of surviving surgery. Twenty years and many operations later, she remains his patient.

"I found out I had a pituitary tumor in December of 1978 and you know something, I was the very first patient of the young doctor who diagnosed it. He said I was lucky, because there was a doctor here who was one of the few who would actually operate in cases like mine. I went as soon as I could.

"When I saw him, I almost didn't believe he was the doctor. He wasn't like any doctor I had met in Oklahoma. He had this long hair, and he wore a silk shirt that was unbuttoned halfway down his chest. And he wore all these gold chains, layered. I almost walked out. But then he started talking. Within thirty minutes I was convinced that he was the doctor for me.

"What I liked was that he was straightforward. On that very first visit he said he would operate, but there was only a fifty-fifty chance that I would get out of the operating room alive. He also went down a long list of other things that could happen to me, including being blind or paralyzed.

"The strange thing was, the more he talked about the details, the less worried I was. I could tell that he was very confident about what he could do. And the alternative—not having the operation—would have meant that I would have definitely died. From that moment on I was never afraid. I don't know why, exactly, but there was something about his manner that made me feel like I was in the best hands and it was going to be all right.

·   ·   ·

"The other thing that I like about Stanley is that he's very tough when it comes to protecting his patients. He does not want you to suffer any more pain than you have to. That feeling is in his soul, and he will go out of his way to make sure you don't have any more pain. When I went to the hospital for my operation, I noticed that almost everything on the top of my chart—my name, age, address—all the information was wrong. It sort of upset me. If they couldn't get that right, then how could I be sure they would take care of me right? I said, 'I'm going home.'

"No sooner did I say that then Stanley comes marching down the hall as mad as a bat. He said to me, 'You pick a hospital. I'll send you there and we'll do the operation.' I picked another hospital and he did just what he said.

"On other times, he has told the hospital that I don't have to come in the night before an operation. He says that he will not require his patients to spend the money staying overnight in a hospital bed when they can come the morning of the operation. I've also seen him tell nurses to get their pocketbooks and leave when he saw that my chart wasn't being kept carefully. He said, 'Your notes are what I depend on to tell me how she's doing. If you can't do that right, then get out.'

"It may sound like he's harsh, but he's really only trying to get the best for me. I know that; and if that means that everyone in the hospital snaps to attention when he comes 'round, then that's okay with me.

"Of course, the people who are on his team, who go into surgery with him, all know that he is the best and so are they. They work very closely and very smoothly. They also recognize that you are a person, not just an open brain lying there. I bumped into one of his nurses one day and she said hello to me. I didn't know who it was until she told me. But she remembered me, not my tumor or my brain, but me.

"I've been a real challenge, like a special project for Stanley. He's told me that. He's said he's just not giving up on me. In that first operation they took out a tumor that was so big he needed both hands to hold it. I had radiation therapy, and I've needed to go back several times to have the damage that's been caused by the radiation repaired.

"Every time, he is the same. He doesn't have someone else prep you; he does it. He shaves your head and he talks to you while he does it. After the operation, he comes in every morning that I'm in the hospital and wakes me up. We talk and he explains what is scheduled for me today. He tells me exactly what they are supposed to do, and he says that if they try to do anything else to me I should call him and he'll make them stop.

"When I say that I have never been afraid, even when he was going into my brain, I mean it. I can joke with him about it. I call him the alien from hell that takes over people's brains.

"He laughs. But the truth is, I wasn't always so confident that things would work out. I would have been very scared before I met him. But he taught me how to not be afraid. By watching him and listening to him, I learned how to be tough, how to take care of me. That's probably the most important thing I've gotten from him, and it was probably the thing I needed the most at the time."

NATALIE HARTMAN, PATIENT

Lavonna Saul is the mother of Natalie Hartman who, in 1980, was born with cerebral palsy, hydrocephaly—fluid swelling her cranium—and spina bifida. As is typical with spina bifida, many of the nerves that would normally run down the spinal column were instead protruding from a hole in Natalie's back. The initial surgery, to repair the opening and reattach nerves, lasted twelve hours. Dozens of smaller operations followed.

"When Natalie was born, they wouldn't even let me hold her because any jostling might have broken the sack that held all the nerves. She would have gotten an infection and probably died right away. But I was still in denial about how serious it all was.

"The first time I met Dr. P. he told me I had a choice to make—operate or let her die. I thought, 'Who does this guy think he is telling me there's something this seriously wrong with my baby?' But as he talked, I started to accept it. Stanley is very calm, very factual. He gave me all the information, but he didn't try to influence my decision. That's the way he is. He gives you all the information, then you have to be tough, strong like him.

"When he came out of the operating room he said that it went very well. He had been able to reattach a lot of the nerves. But we weren't in the clear at all. In the next nine months he had to put seven different shunts into her brain to drain the fluid from the hydrocephaly.

"During that time when we were going through so many operations, Dr. P. let me call him at home whenever I had a question. When I didn't call for a while, he'd get in touch with me just to check on Natalie and see how she was doing. With Stanley, you are not a patient with a problem. You are a person struggling through something very difficult. He understands and he wants to help with your struggle.

"Natalie's father and I got divorced pretty soon after she was born. Since then she's had twenty-seven operations, and every time we go back to Dr. Pelofsky. Natalie is now eighteen years old. She's got a certificate qualifying her to work as a medical assistant and a medical transcriptionist. Stanley has told her that she's got a job in his office when she's ready.

"In all this time I've learned a lot about Dr. Pelofsky. He's a pretty artsy guy. He's gone through a long-hair phase, a hippie look, GQ, and now he's dressing like Sean Connery. But what's inside of him has never changed. He is our Earth Angel. And even if Natalie never needs to have surgery again, we're holding on to him. He's in our family now."

DOCTOR

Born in Brooklyn in 1941, Stanley Pelofsky was a street kid who learned early how to fight. He attended Erasmus Hall High School, where he was steered toward a course in automotive repair. One of his most vivid school memories is of a guidance counselor who, upon hearing Pelofsky's dream of becoming a doctor replied, "Don't make me laugh."

Dr. Pelofsky's earliest professional role model was a disheveled allergist named Dr. Messer, whom he describes as "the lost Marx brother." As Pelofsky recalls, Dr. Messer provided him little relief for his chronic sinusitis, and he found many of the treatments un-comfortable. However, Dr. Messer was a warm, down-to-earth human being, in the Yiddish vernacular, a mensch. "He treated me like he cared, like I was a real person. He liked me, and I liked him. I never missed an appointment."

Stanley Pelofsky is a small, wiry man with dark hair and blue eyes. He is so full of energy that he practically vibrates as he talks. He regularly performs operations that, in Dr. Messer's day, could only be imagined. However, along with the rewards of repairing potentially fatal aneurysms and removing deadly tumors comes a high level of risk associated with such heroic, last-chance surgeries.

"As far as I'm concerned, my effectiveness really depends on my relationship with my patients. They are the ones who keep you on your toes. They teach you everything. The most important lesson, which you learn over and over, is to be ready for the new, the unexpected. That's what I love about my work. It really is exciting and challenging every day.

"I can give you an extreme example of this from a long time ago. It was during Vietnam. I was a new general medical officer assigned to the First Marine Division in Da Nang. I wasn't even a neurosurgeon, really. Anyway, they bring in this soldier who had been fooling around with another Marine. They had accidentally set off this grenade launcher and the grenade had gone into his eye, lodged in the socket, but it hadn't exploded.

"I was pretty nervous, but everyone told me there was no danger of this thing going off when I operated. My boss, the senior surgeon, tells me, 'Stan, you go ahead and get started with this. I'll join you. When I went in to see this fellow he was really

calm. We just talked about what was going to happen. I told him
that I was going to take off his forehead in order to get at the
grenade. I told him he would lose the eye.

"I'll never forget what he told me. He said, 'Doc, you're
number one. I'm here. I know I'm getting the best there is. I
trust you.'

"I realized then that I was this young man's doctor, his father,
his friend, everything. And with this ease, this grace, he had just
put it all in my hands. I also noticed that they were building a
wall of sandbags around the operating room. Obviously they had
lied to me about the fact that this thing could explode. But the
important thing was that we both stay calm and be confident that
it was going to work out okay. We couldn't give in to being
afraid, because then we couldn't do what we had to do.

"The operation was actually pretty straightforward. They
brought in this special box for me to put the round in after I got
it out, then they rushed it outside. It never did go off. When the
Marine came out of the anesthesia I told him that there had been
some frontal lobe damage and he had lost the eye. He said that he
knew that, and that he thought the whole thing was a success.

"We felt very close after going through that together. We
wrote to each other for four or five years after that. He reinforced
something that has stayed with me ever since. In this specialty,
where you are in there under extreme circumstances operating
on someone's brain, often when it's life or death, you have to just
believe in yourself, in your skills, and go do it.

"I never lose sight of how amazing the brain is, and the risks I
am taking. Just think about what it takes for the brain to produce

a great artist, a Modigliani. Every time I operate I am aware that it is the essence of the person. But when there is a tumor of the brain or an aneurysm you have no choice; and the patients who come to me are giving me their ultimate trust. Because of that I am very truthful. I will not cheat them by holding back information.

"But before we even get to that, I sit down and listen to what the patient is hoping will be the outcome. It's easy, really. I say, 'How can I help you?' Then I shut up. Ninety percent of the people will tell you within two minutes exactly what their expectations are.

"With the other 10 percent, you need to make more effort. I use one technique that almost always works. I ask the person to tell me something that they have been trying to tell a doctor but haven't been able to. That's when you hear about bladder and bowel problems and sexual dysfunction. One older woman I operated on told me that what she wanted most was to recover the control of her bladder function. She had never discussed it with anyone. When that happened, she was completely happy with the surgery. She told me, privately, that the best thing was that she didn't have to wear a diaper anymore.

"Even though there's a lot you can do, you have to remind your patients and their families that you are not God. You are not in complete control of what will happen.

"I remind myself of this all the time by remembering a younger woman I operated on in the mid 1970s. She had an aneurysm in the back of the brain about the size of a marble. The aneurysm was going to burst sometime soon, with the result being death or worse, her suffering incredible brain damage. That's why there was really no option but to operate. And she was a good candidate for a pretty successful outcome. The family met with me and they said, 'We trust in you and God to pull us through.'

"Well, when I got into the surgery and reached the aneurysm, I could see the blood swirling around inside it. The aneurysm itself was tissue-paper thin, very fragile. As I exposed it, it just burst. I wasn't even close to it, but it ruptured and bled. She went into cardiac arrest and though we got her started again, she never recovered. She died.

"Her family could see what happened on my face when I came out of surgery. That's one reason you always tell the truth. People know it, anyway. They accepted what happened because I had been honest with them and told them what was possible. But she had four children and a lovely husband, and every time I am doing an operation like that I remember her. I had connected with that family and it really affected me.

"We learn a lot from our mistakes, especially if we are attached to our patients. And of course you get attached, if you are at all honest with people. You see them as human beings, not a procedure to be done. You listen to them, joke with them. You know them. They bake you apple pies and bring them by to surprise you. It's really quite wonderful.

"But this can get you in trouble in ways that you'd never expect, though. It happened with one of those apple pie families. The patient was a woman who had a cervical disk problem that we repaired. She worked at the social security administration and she was very, very eager to get back to work. She called me a week or two before I said she could go and insisted it was okay. Then she showed up at the office with this apple pie and pleaded with me. I took the bribe. She went to work. Her office was in the Murrah Building and she died in the bombing.

"Don't get the idea that my practice is all these difficult outcomes and problems. It's not at all. Even though a lot of patients are mine only when they have one operation, others are with me a long time and working with them is very rewarding.

"There's this young woman Natalie, who came to me when she was very young. She has cerebral palsy. I must have operated on her a dozen times over the years. We even implanted nerves in her spinal cord. Her mother, Lavonna, raised her by herself. They battled everything together, but without help. I became their ally. In a few weeks she's going to graduate from computer school. I couldn't be happier if she was my own child.

"As a whole, my patients have taught me that I must be a human being first, and then a doctor. I have to connect with them and make sure they see I recognize them as individuals. I think about my parents in Brooklyn, all the people I care about. My patients are no different. They are like family who trust me to take care of them.

"When I talk to young doctors I tell them that they must look at themselves realistically. Are they arrogant? Are they stuck-up? Are they abrasive? Are they condescending? If they are, then they are useless. I say, 'Go get a personality. Or go get some psychotherapy. Do something to get over yourself.' This is my opinion. I'm not God. I could be wrong. But I don't think I am. People want a doctor who's a human being first."

Hope and Science

⌣

Anthony Rothschild, M.D., 45,
psychiatry, Worcester, Massachusetts

Irving Brudnick, 70,
businessman, Weston, Massachusetts

⌣

PATIENT

Irving Brudnick was in his first year of medical school at Tulane University when he suffered his initial crippling bout of depression. He was just eighteen years old at the time, and until then his family and friends never considered he would be anything but a doctor. But the morbid thoughts, overwhelming anxiety, and obsession with death that came with acute depression changed everything. He dropped out of school, went into business, and struggled to build a life.

For nearly forty years Brudnick sought help from a variety of therapists, none of whom provided much relief. When his analyst of many years finally retired, he was referred to Dr. Rothschild. He was enrolled in one of the first trials of a new class of drugs called SSAIs (Selective Seratonin Reuptake Inhibitor).

"I was seeing my first doctor when I first met my wife. I came to him and told him I loved this girl but I was very worried about making her put up with someone with my kind of problems. He said, 'Don't worry. But don't tell her anything. Get married. Start a family. Then these episodes of depression will stop.'

"Of course they didn't. My wife would just see me withdraw, get all silent, and sit alone. She didn't know what was wrong. She thought it was her. Eventually I told her what it was, and I said I would understand if she left me, because no one should have to put up with it. But she just looked at me and said she was going to stand by me. She loved me, and that was it. It was a tremendous relief.

"The next time I felt that much weight lifted off my shoulders was many years later when I was referred to Tony Rothschild. First he explained the whole thing about the importance of serotonin in the brain and its effect on neurotransmitters. Then he gave me hope, because he said the research was pointing to some pharmaceutical solutions. But the real important thing was him telling me it was not my fault. And the way he explained the science made it clear that he was right about that.

"Besides trying the drugs, we did psychotherapy, but it was different. We started identifying things that happened, things in my life, that seemed to trigger these episodes. We then looked for ways to avoid them, or to react to them in a more constructive way. Tony respected my strengths. He never failed to return a phone call, and that made me feel like I was actually important to him.

"He also understood how I felt about certain things, like becoming dependent on drugs. I had terrible anxiety once, but another doctor had warned me about never taking more than two pills a day. I finally told Tony that I wasn't taking more than that because of this warning. Well, he said that he knew me well enough to know I wouldn't get in trouble like that. He told me to take another pill, and not worry about it. 'I'm not in the suffering business,' he said. That made me feel a lot better.

"At other times when I was in the middle of a really painful episode of depression, I would be the one who might suggest the hospital or using electroshock because I just wanted some relief. He would listen and he would say, 'Well, we could do that.' But then I'd keep talking and it would be clear that I was really making these suggestions to show how bad I felt. He knew I didn't really want to go in the hospital or have shock treatment. Eventually he'd say, 'Do you want to gut it out for another week?' I'd take on the challenge and knowing that he had faith in me, that he believed I could do it, helped make it possible. Acute depression episodes are self-limiting. They always break. Tony would help me get through it until they did.

"I have always felt that Tony understood me specifically and took care of me in a way that was unique to me. One of the most important things was helping me understand that I have a medical condition, and it's not because of my personality or lack of willpower. We developed the kind of relationship that allowed me to believe him completely when he said this was the case.

"Once I asked him, 'Tony, am I going to be on these drugs all my life?' He said, 'Irv, would a diabetic person on insulin worry about that question if they knew it was keeping them alive?' The answer was, 'Of course not.' I understand that. There's no shame in having this depression, and there's nothing wrong with taking the medication that makes it better. Once someone explains it to you in such a practical, scientific way, it makes it much easier to accept and, to accept yourself the way you are. That's a gift."

DOCTOR

Anthony Rothschild's fascination with the biological and social factors in depression began while he was an undergraduate at Princeton. After medical school at the University of Pennsylvania, a residency in Boston led to work in some of the first trials of modern anti-depression medications. After his formal education, he developed a practice focused primarily on the treatment of depression with a combination of drugs and psychotherapy. He has resisted the movements that have recently divided psychiatry into camps favoring drug treatment or talking therapy.

Born in 1953, Rothschild was raised on Long Island during the postwar boom years. His father was a publishing executive.

His mother was a nursery school teacher and a volunteer in services for the blind. He says that his ability to relate with patients was not something he learned in medical school but rather, a gift from his parents.

"A lot of therapists think they are supposed to be distant, a blank slate. I'm the opposite. When I'm with a patient I literally try to put myself in their position, to feel just what they are feeling. This means I'm opening myself up to some pretty powerful emotions. Usually I can handle it without any problem, but every once in a while there's a patient who really gets to me. That's the risk you take when you try to connect at such a deep level.

"The patient I'm talking about was a woman who had been referred to me from Massachusetts General Hospital. She had gone up to the thirty-fourth floor of the Harbor Towers apartments in Boston, where her parents had an apartment, and jumped off. She had planned it and carried it out. But she had failed. She had lived. And now she was in a lot of physical pain to go along with her depression.

"At first in our sessions all she could do was sit and cry and say, 'I want to die.' When I listened to her, I could really feel how terrible she felt. She was really hopeless and I found myself asking her, quite seriously, if there was anything she could think of that made her life worth living. The truth was, I could feel how desperate she was, and I couldn't really think of anything else to say. She could see that. She could tell I understood and I think that really made a difference.

"That empathy helped get her through the first few weeks while the medications started to work. Gradually we began to talk about the things in her life that were so troubling, like her chronic pain, her marriage. She explained to me that she had felt that if there was no hope, that her life was always going to be as painful as it felt when she made that jump, then she didn't want to live anymore. I was able to show her that she had a medical condition—delusional depression—and that it could be treated.

"The truth is that depression is a very serious medical condition—often a fatal one—and not a sign that there's something wrong or bad about an individual person. In fact, I spend a lot of time talking to people whose disease could have very well killed them. Studies have shown that more than half of those who do die by suicide have actually seen some kind of doctor in the month before. Unfortunately the doctor doesn't see what's happening. At the same time the person has no friend or family to talk to, no one to give them hope. Hope is the next thing I try to establish. If you show a patient that you truly understand what they are feeling, that it is a medical condition, and that there is something that can be done, then you have the basic foundation for a good relationship.

"When I first started seeing Irving he had been through years and years of talking therapy. He had this kind of ruminative depression, where he felt overwhelming guilt. He felt shame and responsibility for what was wrong, like he was somehow to blame. It was very painful for me to just tap into what he was feeling, it was that strong.

"But very early on, I said something that obviously made a very big impression on him. I said, 'This is a pretty common syndrome, and it responds well to medication and psychotherapy.'

"He interrupted me and said, 'So, is it my fault or not?'

"I really was surprised by his question. I told him that of course it wasn't his fault. It's a medical problem, and it can be taken care of by medical treatment. That simple statement really forged the relationship because, as I learned later, he had always been feeling that his depression was somehow a reflection of his character; that he was weak or something. In fact, as anyone who gets to know him can see, Irving has a very strong character. He responds very well to challenges, and he has a very supportive family. Those strengths and his approach to problems are something I try to use for his benefit.

"Talking therapy and SSAI drugs have helped Irving, but the acute episodes of depression still occur. There have been several times when the question of whether we should put him in the hospital for a while has come up. Hospitalization can speed up a patient's treatment, and while I'm a little reluctant to do it with anyone, I'll recommend it when necessary. But for Irving it has a lot of negative connotations, as if it reflects a failure. So when it seems like he's close, we talk about it and I give him the pros and cons, but we hold the decision. Invariably he has gotten better before needing to go in, and I think that has to do with his own resources. Our relationship is close enough that I know how he can respond to the challenge of perhaps going into the hospital and get better more quickly.

"But while I try to make collaborative decisions with patients, I never forget that they are turning to me for expertise. Irving has sometimes made changes in his medications on his own. A lot of patients do that. When they do, I raise objections because I need to know what's happening. If we are a team working on their recovery I have to have the truth. Openness is very important, because people can do things with medications that are dangerous. If someone wants to combine Prozac and St. John's wort for example, I object immediately.

"Open, honest relationships mean that a patient can rely on me even when their disease is making it difficult for them to accept what I am saying. The classic example is the man whose wife called me recently to say she thought his mania was kicking up. He hadn't had an episode in ten years. But all of a sudden he wasn't sleeping very much, he was working around the clock, he was a little argumentative and he was talking a little faster than normal. All these things are signs that the medication needs to be adjusted, but many people who are in the early stage of mania refuse to acknowledge what other people see happening.

"Fortunately our relationship was good enough that he trusted me. I was also able to tell him, 'I remember that the last time this happened you got arrested for drunk driving, wound up in a hospital, and lost your job.' He came in to see me right away.

"A lot of people, friends, or even colleagues in medicine, say things to me like, 'How can you spend so much time with people who are in so much pain?' Well, the truth is that it's very gratifying to help people who are suffering and see them get better. I've had patients who have told me that depression is worse than cancer, worse than anything, because it so pervades their lives. When they finally get help, the change is dramatic. I don't think there's a more grateful patient population in any other specialty."

The Confidence Man

∾

Fredric Frigoletto, M.D., 66, obstetrician/gynecologist,
Boston, Massachusetts

Anne Bitler, 62, homemaker, Hudson, New Hampshire,
and Melissa Sarner, 30, dentist,
Franklin, Massachusetts

∾

ANNE BITLER, PATIENT

When she first walked into Dr. Frigoletto's office in 1969, Anne Bitler was thirty-three years old, and desperate to save her unborn baby. She had been referred because Frigoletto was among the few doctors known to be expert at intra-uterine transfusions [blood transfusions given before the baby is born]. If anyone could deal with the RH incompatibility affecting her pregnancy, he could.

During weekly visits and several transfusions, Mrs. Bitler forged a close relationship with her new physician. Even before her baby was born—premature but healthy—she decided he would become her regular gynecologist. They have remained doctor and patient ever since.

"I was really scared. I mean, I had already been told that it was very possible I would lose the baby. I had been sent to Dr. Frigoletto as a kind of last resort. But you know, from the very beginning he was so kind and so positive. He had so much confidence that it gave me confidence. I think that was the thing that impressed me the most at first. He was sure that things would work out, and it made me sure too.

"The procedure made me quite nervous. They passed a long needle through my abdomen, into the uterus, and into the baby. He used an X ray to guide him, but it was really a pretty demanding job. But he explained everything beforehand—the risks and the benefits—and he answered every question, including when I asked what he would do in my situation. A lot of doctors don't take time for all these questions. They act like you are dumb for asking them. I have never felt that from Dr. Frigoletto. By the time the transfusion started I felt like I was prepared and ready.

"In the years since, he has always been my gynecologist. Twice we've discovered cysts in my breasts during an exam. In both cases they were benign, but you don't know that when they are discovered. The way he handled it was so sensitive. The second time, when the mammogram showed something more suspicious, he followed up on my case very closely. He knew how frightened I was, so he called me before I saw the surgeon and said he wanted to hear from me right after my appointment. Then he called again. It was a frightening time for me, and I know he was responding to that, to my feelings, not just my problem.

"I guess that's the thing a lot of women want when they are seeing a gynecologist. I mean, the truth is, no one likes those exams. As you get older, it gets worse. But with Dr. Frigoletto you feel nothing but respect. It's almost like he treats you as a colleague. And you are never just a body part. You are a person, and you matter."

MELISSA SARNER, PATIENT

The daughter of Anne Bitler, Melissa Sarner was the RH-factor baby who received transfusions in-utero from Dr. Frigoletto. When it was time to choose her own obstetrician, to deliver her first baby, Sarner did not consider any other doctor.

"He doesn't just shake your hand. He takes it gently in his and then holds it for a moment while you talk. I like that. But then, it is the kind of thing you expect from him. He makes you feel like he has nothing else on his mind, and nothing that he has to do next. He is there, focused on you.

"In my family, Dr. Frigoletto is very respected. I mean, he was literally responsible for me being here on this Earth. He jokes now and tells me that I was born green, like the Incredible Hulk. But it was no joke. No one could say for sure that I was going to live, but he was dedicated. He helped me survive and he saw my mother through it.

"A woman's relationship with an obstetrician or gynecologist is unusual. I mean, everyone feels uncomfortable at first. Sometimes you wonder if the people going into this kind of medicine really like women at all. But not Dr. Frigoletto. You definitely get the idea that he just loves it, even after all these years. I can complain about morning sickness and he listens. And when I had some bleeding early in my pregnancies he saw me right away. He was very reassuring. He didn't promise anything without the test results or anything, but he let me know that everything was going to be all right.

"When you can trust your doctor, trust his judgment and trust that he's really listening to you, that's everything. I know he's there, focused on me and my baby and nothing else. And I know that he's got all the experience and knowledge to help me. Whatever it is, he's seen it, and he can handle it. It's really great to know that."

DOCTOR

As a boy, Fredric Frigoletto often stopped by his father's dental office on the way home from school. Born in 1933, young Fredric watched his father coax his patients through treatments that were

often painful. It was his first glimpse of the healing power of relationships.

As a medical student, Frigoletto sneaked into Boston City
Hospital to see, for the first time, a baby being born. Later, during an eight-week summer program at Framingham Hospital, he
traded with other students so that he could spend each of the
four two-week rotations in obstetrics. By the end of that summer he knew he wanted to dedicate his life's work to helping
mothers bring infants into the world. During his practice, which
began in 1960, he witnessed a revolution in how this is done.
Today he heads a large group practice that counts, among its
members, a team of nurse midwives.

"In the early years, women still gave birth under what was called
a twilight anesthesia. But having a baby was still frightening for
a woman, and the doctor's support was very important to see
her through it. Then came epidural anesthetics and the women's
movement, which meant that mothers and fathers would be
much more involved. I guess I was prepared for this change because I've always been a great believer in giving patients as much
choice and control as possible. My bottom line is, as long as you
won't hurt yourself, as long as it's not dangerous, I'll support you.

"I think that understanding that you are there to be supportive and provide medical expertise, is the key. Add a real attentive-
ness to each patient during a visit, and real respect, and you have
a good relationship. I still see many patients that I first treated
twenty or twenty-five years ago. In gynecology, where the patient has to be made to feel comfortable, patients tend to stay
with a doctor who has done it right.

"One of those long-term patients is a woman I saw first in the late 1960s. Back then the treatment of the unborn child in-utero was just starting. Intra-uterine fetal blood transfusions for babies that had an RH incompatibility were just beginning. The patient I saw had already lost at least one child to this problem and was now pregnant with another. I was enlisted to help with the transfusion. Back then you did everything. You gathered the equipment—the tubing and syringes—and you did all the patient visits. The procedures were done at seven- to ten-day intervals. Every time I saw her I knew that the possibility of disaster was hanging over her. I didn't ignore that fact. But I also made it clear that we would do everything to make sure disaster didn't occur.

"That woman was a very private person and very quiet, but intense. She's been my patient ever since. And now that baby who I treated in-utero is also a patient of mine about to have her first baby.

"In cases like that first one, you are working together on a very serious problem and the relationship is kind of built out of that effort. In a more regular circumstance, say when a woman is coming in for her first exam, it's my job to understand what her expectations are. These encounters are full of inner emotions, and, understandably, some anxiety.

"I focus pretty intently on taking both a social history and medical history. I take my time and I listen, because in that infor- mation are some important clues to what a patient is feeling. Few patients are going to put everything out there for you. You have to intuit some things, and use your experience to ask the right questions.

"With pregnancies you often have to establish a good relationship with the husband, or partner, who is going to be the coach. It's kind of a triangular relationship and there's a lot to be learned by observing it. I recently had a patient whose husband seemed antagonistic with me and very controlling with his wife. Even as we were meeting, he was giving her instructions and trying to impress me with all that he knew. That's the kind of thing you can see if you are attuned to everything going on in the relationship.

"There are a lot of other things you encounter that are outside medical issues, per se. I mean, we have patients who are homeless or are using drugs. Before we send a mother home we have to know: Is there money for food? Do you have a car seat? Is there really a home to go to at all? We do our level best to help people with all these problems. Of course, they are adults, and they have autonomy. But if you have that relationship, there's often something you can do.

"If there is one thing I think I could share it's that you must never be a robot. Don't let yourself fall into a pattern of treating everyone the same. Patients are all individuals who need to be listened to and respected. I have never been sued by a patient, and I think that's because they know that I am always paying attention to their needs and doing my best for them specifically. No one is treated like a number.

"Then of course, there's always the unexpected. Sometimes it has nothing to do with a patient. Once I was in my office and I heard this crashing in the waiting room, like chairs being tipped over. When I got outside, I find two men fighting. One is the husband of a patient. His arm is in a sling because the week before he lost some fingers in a snowblower. The other is a one-legged man with no crutches who has a gun. He's mad because the first guy had splashed him with slush when he was driving up for his appointment.

"Anyway, when I come out, they run out onto the sidewalk. While I'm calling the police, a woman who is in the parking lot watching all of this has a heart attack.

"Now, as hard as that is to believe, there's more. Two days later I see a patient. She says she was in court the day before and heard a one-legged man tell the judge that I had beat him up. We had a real good laugh about that. She knew it couldn't have been true, because she knew me well. But we sure had a laugh."

Science at Your Service

❧

Shelley Giebel, M.D., 36,
gynecologist, Temple, Texas

Ashley Tongate, 7, student, whose mother is
Denise Tongate, 34, a medical technician, Buckholts, Texas

❧

PATIENT

Seven-year-old Ashley Tongate's medical odyssey began when she was two years old and ended when she was six. In that time her mother, Denise Tongate, took her from doctor to doctor until she finally found Shelley Giebel, M.D., a gynecologist, in Temple, Texas.

Denise Tongate

"Ashley had had a lot of ear infections when she was very little and had been treated with a lot of antibiotics. The real problem started after that, when she was two, and she just started squirming all over the place.

"The main symptom was that she couldn't sit still, couldn't really sit down at all. She also complained about going to the bathroom. She said it was uncomfortable, and she would go a long time without using the toilet at all.

"When we first brought her to a pediatrician he examined her a little bit and said she might be a little red down there, but that it was nothing but slight irritation. He said, 'Put her in a baking soda bath; that will relieve the discomfort, and she'll be alright.'

"Well, we must have tried baths for over a year and it never really got much better. It's hard to explain to you just how uncomfortable Ashley was. I would try to have her go to the bathroom before school and she was miserable. At school she just fidgeted and squirmed all day, driving the teachers crazy. Eventually it got so that she tried not to drink anything at all, because she didn't want to urinate. I mean, she was getting dehydrated.

"I thought there was something seriously wrong, so I asked for a referral to a gynecologist. I was told that was ridiculous, that she was too young and there was no reason for that. They sent me to a urologist instead, and that was when things got even more frustrating. He ordered a bunch of tests, but he never really even looked at Ashley or talked to me. I could tell that the tests were being done just to get rid of us, to buy him some time because he thought we might just go away.

"When the tests came back negative the doctor told us that it was all in Ashley's mind. There was nothing wrong with her, but maybe she was hyperactive. He referred me to a psychiatrist and said he thought we should try putting her on Ritalin. When I started to cry out of frustration, the doctor just walked out.

"After all of this I tried to think of who might help us. I knew Dr. Giebel's husband because I work in the hospital lab where they do stress tests, and he's a cardiologist. It was really out of desperation that I called her.

"The most amazing thing happened when I called her office. First the receptionist talked to me and heard the basic story. Then she put me on hold for a minute. When she came back on she asked me to tell it again, with a little more detail. She listened very carefully and asked a lot of questions. At some point I started to think it wasn't the same person that I had started talking to. So I asked, 'Who is this?'

"She said, 'Why, this is Dr. Giebel.'

"I couldn't believe it. Here was a doctor I didn't know, who wasn't even in my network, getting right on the phone to hear the story and ask all these questions. Then she asked me if I could get Ashley to her office right away. I said that I had to get her out of school, but that I would. She saw us as soon as we got to her office. She figured out what was wrong that day, and in two or three days Ashley was feeling much better. She's been better ever since.

"What did Dr. Giebel do that the others didn't? She took us seriously. She respected both me and Ashley."

DOCTOR

Born and raised in Houston, Dr. Giebel received her medical education at Texas A&M and performed her residency in gynecology at the Mayo Clinic in Rochester, Minnesota. She began practice in an obstetrics and gynecology group, but recently opened a solo practice restricted to gynecology. Both her father and her husband are physicians.

"I could tell on the phone that both Ashley and Denise were suffering a lot with this. I mean think about it. You can't sit down or use the bathroom comfortably and this goes on for years. You go to these doctors and they don't help you. It's embarrassing and upsetting for you. If you are the mother you feel terrible that you can't help your child. It was an awful situation.

"And the worst part was, it doesn't take a mental giant to figure out what is going on if you listen to the symptoms or do the right kind of exam. Ashley had a combination of a yeast infection, contact dermititis, and bladder infection.

"I suppose that a lot of doctors wouldn't think of a yeast infection because Ashley was so young. It is very rare. And I think a lot of doctors would refuse to send her to a gynecologist because they believe she's too young or they don't really listen to the symptoms.

"But remember, she had received all those antibiotics, which sets someone up for a subsequent yeast infection. And the symptoms she described were classic. All you have to do is listen to them, believe that what you are being told is the truth, and you get the diagnosis. The other part was doing the exam. A lot of doctors might be reluctant to do it, but if you establish a caring relationship with a child, it works out fine. Ashley wanted to feel better. She trusted that I wanted that for her too, so it was not difficult.

"My father was an endocrinologist who absolutely loved his work. I grew up going to the hospital with him, playing with plastic kidneys and other organs. On Sunday mornings he would give us lectures and he'd give us little quizzes like, 'I have a patient whose glucose is 800. What's wrong with her?' And I would shout, 'Diabetes!'

"When I got into high school and college, I worked in his office. He taught me how to draw blood, and he would invite me in the room to observe whenever he had an interesting case. The science really fascinated me, but I also could see that he cared very deeply for his patients. Both of those things attracted me to medicine: the intellectual part and the connection with the people.

"The most amazing thing about obstetrics and gynecology is that you are dealing with people in some of the most extreme circumstances a person ever faces. Once, in residency, within the space of thirty minutes I delivered a beautiful baby for this very happy couple and then had to tell another pregnant woman that the baby had died in her womb. You learn to rely on everything you have ever experienced in life, everything that lets you connect with people, to get through situations like that. Mostly it comes down to respecting them and what they are going through. It's an honor to be there with them.

"I learned a lot about working with patients in residency. A lot of what I learned was seeing very good medicine along with very obvious examples of how not to interact with people. I remember one very graphic example. There was this one young woman, very beautiful, who had a very unusual genital abnormality which she had come a long way to have fixed. I was in the exam room with this very prominent expert who was going to do it. When he looked at her he made this awful face like he was disgusted and some kind of comment like he couldn't believe what he was seeing. I stood up by her head, holding her hand and apologizing for what the other doctor was doing and saying.

"In my training I realized that we had allowed society to label us as doctors, to put us in what was supposedly a position of high esteem, but deny us the right to be down-to-earth human beings. The profession had accepted it, and concluded that we couldn't handle it if we were really openly connected with the patients.

"But the truth is the opposite. It's much easier to deal with things if you let yourself feel what is going on. You also get much more information from your patients if you reveal yourself as a person. I have a child and people know it. I share with them what it's like to balance everything in life. Patients also want to know if what they are experiencing is normal. If I have been through the same thing, I tell them.

. . .

"There are also a lot of little things you can do so that your practice reflects your respect for your patients. The first thing I did was I called this 'our practice' when I'm talking with the staff rather than 'my practice.' They feel like this is their office, and they respond very carefully to the patients from the moment they first call the office. We don't make people wait in our office. I take all of the history myself. And I give every patient a full hour for the first visit. This is a sacred relationship we are forming and I don't rush it.

"There are other things we do. We never have the patient undress and wait for us. We talk first about what we're going to do and then I leave while they change. We have only cloth gowns, and we always have some in very large sizes for big women. They are so grateful for that. We use several different sizes of speculum, and they are specially designed so that women don't have to shift all over the table into the most embarrassing positions possible. Every thing is warmed before it is used. We have little soft covers on the stirrups. We have only cloth sheets on the examining table, not that roll of paper. These are all obvious things that show we respect our patients, but not everyone does it.

"We're in Texas, which is a pretty conservative state socially, so I use a printed questionnaire to give people the opportunity to tell me about problems they may feel uncomfortable about raising face-to-face. With this form I've actually learned about several women's history of sexual abuse.

"I also do not judge patients. Gynecology has a lot to do with people's sexual behavior and values. I've had patients come in—adults—who were denied prescriptions for birth control by doctors who refuse because the woman isn't married.

. . .

"The most important thing to remember is that being open and respectful to the patients is very rewarding for the doctor. If you practice this way, you find that you have many more positive encounters with people. Ninety-nine percent of the time they will trust you enough to tell you everything you need to know to help them. This is the kind of medicine that makes you realize that you don't do it for the money. You do it because it is meaningful work, and that's more valuable than anything."

Patience for Patients

༄

George Hanna, M.D., 45, cardiologist,
Providence, Rhode Island

John Suchwalko, 41, telephone technician,
North Providence, Rhode Island

༄

PATIENT

At age thirty-four, John Suchwalko thought he was in good health. But after walking up and down the Civil War battlefield in Gettysburg, he came home from his vacation hobbled by a muscle pull. Having last seen a doctor a decade before, he went to the hospital emergency room for care. There he was discovered to have exceedingly high blood pressure and early signs of diabetes. He was referred to Dr. George Hanna.

"My blood pressure was off the charts, but I didn't feel anything. That's why they call it the silent killer. The same was true with my cholesterol. Dr. Hanna said it was the highest he had ever seen. I was also overweight. I was six foot-one, and 255 pounds. I smoked and I didn't get much real exercise.

"The thing that impressed me about Dr. Hanna was that he didn't come down on me real hard. I didn't feel like I had been sent to the vice principal's office and he was wagging a finger in my face saying, 'You better do this' or 'You better do that.'

"Instead, he came across like he was a very knowledgeable friend. He said that I had a pretty high risk of heart attack or stroke, and that if nothing changed I'd probably have to go on insulin. 'You're still a pretty young man. Do you want to see these things happen?'

"When I said that of course I didn't want that, he told me that we could prevent it. We had a lot of work to do, but it could be done. It wasn't impossible. From then on, I was on a diet, I started walking every day, and I came in to his office every two weeks. He would talk to me, encourage me, keep me going. That helped a lot.

"If you want to understand how important it was that Dr. Hanna was so caring, you have to consider what I had been through in the past. I mean, what my family had been through. My father had two strokes, one in 1982 and one in 1986, that came with a heart attack. He was in a coma for nine months and then died. I had an older brother who died in 1985 of a hemorrhage. He was just thirty-three.

"I remember as a kid that my father went to the doctor one day and came home all pissed off. He had had a physical six months before, and the doctor had told him then to lose weight. This time when he went into the office he heard the doctor say to the nurse, 'If he hasn't lost twenty pounds since he was last here, kick him out, because I don't want to see him.' My father left.

"So you can see why I was a little afraid of doctors. I mean, my attitude was that if you didn't feel too bad, then they can either confirm that you aren't very sick or tell you that you've got something terrible that you never expected.

"With Dr. Hanna I didn't get the feeling that this was something impossible to beat. He used a lot of logic and respect, and he showed that he cared about me. His positive approach, and the fact that he was willing to see me every two weeks to help me stay on track made all the difference. I didn't need to be yelled at. I knew I was responsible for helping myself. He just made that a whole lot easier."

DOCTOR

George Hanna was first captivated by the field of medicine as a young boy watching television documentaries of surgical procedures. An uncle who was the doctor in the family also influenced his decision to become a physician. During years of practice, his respect for the patient-physician relationship has grown to match his fascination with the science of medicine.

"I love the science of cardiology. I read everything I can find, and I am fascinated by the progress we make every year. Today you can honestly tell people that there may be a development in the near future that improves their condition. That's very exciting.

"Technical competence, knowing your field, is very important even in relating to patients. They want to know that you are up on top of everything. That's very reassuring. But I have seen some of the best doctors, especially the ones who let everyone else know how smart they are, falter because this affects their relationships with patients and colleagues. This attitude can be destructive.

"As the years go by, you start to understand that the emotional part is very important. I'm not just talking about the patient's feelings, but the doctor's too. I mean, I can't help but get attached to my patients, like they were family members. I wind up being afraid of what might happen to them and I find myself going over and over things in my mind. I'm always wondering if there's one more thing I should try, or something I could do differently.

"In cardiology the patient's lifestyle and attitudes are a very big part of the picture, and the way that you can affect those factors is in the relationship. If you establish trust with someone, get close to them, they will show you what their attitudes are.

"For example, I have had patients who are literally intending to die. It's almost as if they have an inner persecution complex.

Some of them start to talk about dying. The illness is the last drama, the last punishment for them. These are the patients who continue to drink and smoke and do everything wrong for themselves. I know I have to turn them around, or they will make what they believe come true.

"One patient like that—he was in his sixties—really got my attention because I felt that he could live a long time if he just changed a few things. I wound up spending an awful lot of time talking to him, showing him that I cared whether he lived or died, even if he didn't. I would even tell him if I smelled cigarette smoke when I was with him. He knew it was because I cared, and he started to turn around because of it. He moved to Florida a while ago and is doing well. He's no longer my patient but he's still my friend.

"It's not always so easy, and sometimes you have to hang in there a much longer time. Patience was very important with one younger man who came to me because his mother had already lost her husband and one son to heart disease and this son had a cholesterol count of something like 900 and weighed about 300 pounds.

"I saw him every other week to keep close tabs on him, but he didn't improve very much. He was a hockey player, a goalie, and he worked for the phone company. After a while I learned he was going out for beers after the games with his teammates. He said he was going to stop, but even after he did, there wasn't much improvement.

"As time went by, we got close enough for him to admit that he had never stopped drinking and he was unable to do it on his own. I encouraged him to get into Alcoholics Anonymous and he did. But I went a step further. I told him that he could call me any time he wanted a drink and I would talk to him, be there for him. I gave him my phone number and he did use it a few times.

"As you know, there are relapses with alcoholics and he had a few. He lost his job. He lost his health insurance. But I continued to see him. Eventually he got sober and stayed sober. He lost about 120 pounds in eighteen months. He got his job back and is much healthier. And his mother isn't going to lose a second son any time soon.

"The relationship you make with a patient is something that can influence how their medical problems turn out. This is especially true when the condition has something to do with their life choices. When patients want to know why their arteries are clogged, I tell them that it's a lifetime of choices. There are reasons why disease happens, and when they understand it they can start making changes. But the relationship can't be based on me being judgmental or superior acting. It has to be a caring thing.

"If you care, and you demonstrate it, you can build trust with a patient. Some patients come in and they are so skeptical. Often these are very intelligent people who have an hour and a half of questions to ask, and they are testing you every step of the way. Often they do this as a defense, because they are scared. If you show them you have the expertise to understand their problem and treat them, it helps a great deal.

"Being a doctor is stressful. It can be exhausting. But don't let anyone tell you it's not rewarding. The most amazing thing about this is that the doctor-patient relationship is so good for me.

The patients are almost always very nice to me. Even those who I lose, who die, are good to me right to the end. It's like we help each other through it. That's what I think I'd like every doctor to know about the importance of these relationships. It's worth it to put in the time and to let yourself care. It's better for the patients, but in the end, it's a lot better for you, too."

The Pioneer

෴

James Bennett, M.D., 44, urologist,
Atlanta, Georgia

Linda Richardson, 46, insurance executive,
Atlanta, Georgia

෴

PATIENT

Linda Richardson was just thirty-six years old when she began to
suffer from recurrent bladder infections. Initial exams showed
nothing unusual. A year later, her symptoms worsening, she

learned she had bladder cancer. Partial removal of her bladder followed by chemotherapy were not enough. When the cancer recurred, she began looking for a pioneer in urological surgery. That was when she found Dr. Bennett.

"I had been pretty healthy all my life. I had taken care of myself, gone to the doctor for checkups, and I had never had a major illness. I thought I was on top of things. But I now know I was a little naive. I really didn't know how to work with a doctor. I didn't know what my expectations should be and how to assert myself.

"When I was diagnosed with cancer I was only thirty-six. It was very upsetting. A friend recommended I read some books. One of them was *Love, Medicine and Miracles* by Bernie Siegel. Those books gave me the confidence to put my judgment first. They taught me that doctors are very well trained and know their stuff, but we know our own bodies better. We can accept what doctors tell us, but we don't have to let them make decisions for us.

"After the first surgery, the oncologist I went to told me immediately that my whole bladder should have been removed. He predicted that the cancer would come back and it did, in less than a year. I knew that this time they would take the entire thing out, but I also knew that there was some new surgical techniques that might let me avoid having one of those bags on the outside of my body for the rest of my life. At my age, I wanted to avoid that if it was at all possible.

"This kind of operation wasn't something my original urologist had ever done, so my primary care physician sent me to

Dr. Bennett. He had been a pioneer in it and was very experienced with it. When I met with him it was pretty clear to me that he was confident that he could help me, but he wasn't promising miracles. He said, 'I've done many of these operations and I have a good success rate. But I'm not God. I'm not going to be able to give you back what God gave you. But it should be pretty good.'

"He was very confident, which I liked, and very scientific. And he seemed to respect the fact that I had done my research and I had some specific questions about his record, the possible negative outcomes, and my prognosis for the future. We came to an understanding. I was making the decision, and he was going to use his skills to help me the best he possibly could.

"There was another thing that I noticed about Dr. Bennett that was also very important. He seemed to be very aware of who I was, that I was still fairly young, and that this was going to affect my life in a lot of ways. One of the things he did was arrange to have another surgeon there for the operation so they could make the kind of repairs that would allow me to have a normal sex life. When they take out your bladder there's a lot of other tissue that comes out too. He was sensitive to my needs, and I really appreciated that.

"Dr. Bennett is serious about helping people, about using his excellent surgical skills to improve the quality of life for his patients. I guess that's what came through to me. He was really excited about using new techniques, advancing the science, but it was always in order to help people.

"I go back every six months for checkups and everything has been fine for a long time. Recently I went to see him and he told me about this new operation he had done, in another country, where he reconstructed a bladder and then was able to reconnect the urethra in a way that allowed his patient to go to the bathroom normally, without a catheter. He was really excited about the surgical success, his technique. But he was more interested in the fact that he had restored someone to normal. It was about the person, not the medicine, and I liked that a lot."

DOCTOR

The defining moment in James Bennett's life is marked by the wail of a siren and the sight of an ambulance rushing to the scene of an accident. Then just twelve years old, Bennett knew in an instant that someone in his father's logging crew had been injured in the Georgia woods. Soon he would discover that it was his father, and that he had been killed when a tractor overturned.

From the moment of his father's death, Bennett vowed to make a life that was more stable and less dangerous than his father's. The town's only black physician became his mentor, and soon he was determined to become a doctor. "He was very gentle, very understanding, and very much respected by the community," recalls Bennett. "No wonder I wanted to be like him."

"I believe there are scientific answers to every question. We may not have all the answers yet, but they are waiting to be discovered. But I think that for my patients, it's just as important that I recognize that medicine is an art. It's the art of being with people and understanding them, no matter who they are and where they come from. I grew up in rural Georgia. No one in my family had finished school past about the eighth grade. We didn't have indoor plumbing for a long time. So you see, I can relate to just about anyone.

"This is very important in a specialty like urology, which involves a lot of things that people don't want to talk about. You have to make them comfortable. That's why I look at a patient's chart before I go into the room, but I never carry it in with me. I don't take notes while they talk, either. I'll do that later. I don't want anything to come between us. I want them to know I am listening very carefully.

"Obviously urology involves a lot of male patients, and they can be very difficult to get information out of. I mean, most urologists will ask, 'How are you urinating?' The guy will say, 'Fine' and that's it.

"I don't settle for that. I'll give him an example, like, 'Could you write your name in the snow when you pee?' If he says he couldn't do that anymore, I've got some valuable information.

"I also make an effort to get their wives in the room. That will get it out. Once I asked a man to tell me how many times he gets up every night to urinate. He said, 'Never.' Then his wife said, 'What about that jug under the bed?' It turned out that he had been rolling over and peeing into this jug. I would never have thought to ask about something like that specifically, but having his wife present meant I got the information.

"None of this really takes me by surprise. I mean, I learned very early in life that people live in all kinds of ways and have all kinds of habits. I'm here to help all of them, if I can.

.   .   .

"One way you help is by giving them hope. I never take away hope. I also give them as much concrete information—facts—as I can. Some physicians might think this overwhelms patients, but I think it does the opposite. It makes them feel like they understand what's happening to them. A good example of this is the patient with prostate cancer. The absolute truth is that there is not one proven best treatment for it. Once patients understand this, we can discuss all the options and make choices together about what will be done.

"Just being open about the facts helps people a lot. This is really true with impotence. There's some controversy over whether this is a medical problem. I don't have any doubt that it is. How can you place a value on a man's ability to function? Even if you say that the benefit from helping him is solely psychological, what's wrong with that?

"Sexuality is very important to people. I'm not here to judge anyone, or impose my ideas on them. But I do think that if someone wants to be sexual, to express themselves that way, it's part of normal human functioning and I want to help them if I can. This means that I have to be open, too. I've learned a lot about this working with spinal cord injury patients. A lot of what happens sexually takes place in the brain. Even people who are paralyzed can have sex, very enjoyably, if they learn new ways to do it.

"The ability to be open with people, to understand the importance of sexuality, and my interest in the science is a pretty good combination. I think other doctors know my reputation. It's probably why I got the call from the trauma surgeon when one of my patients was in a terrible motor vehicle accident. He had actually had his penis almost burned off. He was not even twenty years old.

"Well, I talked to him for a long time. I acknowledged the trauma he had experienced, but I also gave him hope. We developed a strategy to reconstruct it for him, using what was left as a start. He now has full function, and he has a chance at leading a normal life. I think our relationship, and the confidence we developed in each other, was a big part of it. It wasn't the surgical success that was the most important thing. It was that we helped that young man stay whole as a person with a future."

PART TWO

～

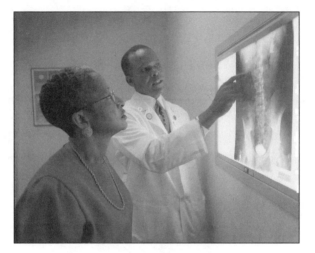

Dr. James Bennett

The
Teachers

～

Dr. Crusader

⤳

Walter M. Bortz III, M.D., 68, gerontologist,
Palo Alto, California

Richard Tuttle, 78, judge,
Mokelumne Hill, California

⤳

PATIENT

Judge Tuttle still hears cases in California state courts and is an
active hiker who, since turning sixty, has climbed Mt. Fuji and

trekked in the Himalayas. He began seeing Dr. Bortz in 1978, at the age of fifty-eight.

"I didn't want a doctor who was going to stand around until I got sick and then decided which kind of operation I needed. I wanted a doctor who was going to actually help me stay away from doctors as much as possible, in other words, one who would help keep me healthy.

"I've got pretty good reason to be concerned about this. My family, the Tuttles, has been in America since the 1600s. Hardly any of the men lived past fifty. My father died at age fifty-nine. My brother at age sixty-four. I wanted to do whatever I could to prevent that from happening to me. I guess you could say that my main health problem is that I've got poor genes, and I wanted some help overcoming that.

"When I met Dr. Bortz I found someone who thought that a lot of what we call aging in this country is actual cultural. It's people deciding to give up on life, to retire and basically quit functioning way too early. I remember when I first saw him I told him that I had the opportunity to go to hike in the Himalayas, but I was concerned about whether I was up to it. He told me that if I kept myself in reasonably good shape there was no reason I couldn't do it. And I did.

"One of the things Dr. Bortz does—sometimes this is subtle and sometimes it is not—is give you examples or role models. He's the first one, obviously. I mean, the man still runs marathons. You go in to see him, and he'll say he ran ten miles in the hills over the weekend. Then he'll tell you about the ninety-two-year-old who was a classmate of his father's at Harvard Medical School who still competes in track and field events.

"Now I can see how some people who are terribly out of condition and have so far to go might not respond to him. But he doesn't tell you that you should run marathons just like him, or that you must run ten miles a weekend. He just tells you that if you don't use your body and your mind that they are going to deteriorate. And that it's almost impossible to use them too much. The rest is up to you.

"Now I'm a person who can relate pretty well to him, and I respond to challenges. When I was seventy-three I told him that I was going to Japan. He said, 'Well, you ought to climb Mt. Fuji if you are over there.'

"Now I wasn't going to be anywhere near Mt. Fuji and I told him so. But afterwards it began to work on me. And don't you know that before I left Japan I paid a cab driver $150 to take me to Mt. Fuji so I could climb it?

"I was very glad that I did. And it happened because of me and because of him. I mean, he knows what kind of person I am and how I'll respond to a challenge. That's part of our relationship. That's a very important part of how he takes care of his patients, the relationship. Other doctors may have all the merit badges that indicate they have technical proficiency, but it's not the same as a relationship.

"I have had some actual medical problems over the years. I had a benign tumor near a testicle, and Dr. Bortz managed to get me the best care available. It was treated with medication and that was it. I also had a minor blood pressure problem, but here again he helped me handle it myself. I had gone into a supermarket and used one of those blood pressure machines and found it was pretty high. Now I like salty things: pretzels, pickles, you name it. He told me to just cut back on the salt and that was enough to bring the blood pressure under control.

"Other than things like that, Dr. Bortz doesn't really prescribe specifically. He just tells you what you need to do if you want to lead a long healthy life. It's up to you to choose how you do it. Sex is a pretty good example of this. He knows I have a healthy sex life, and so he just tells me that it's good for me and that's it. I suppose he might prescribe intercourse if he thought I needed it, but he knows I don't.

"Besides physical activity, Dr. Bortz also advises that you keep your mind active. Until two years ago I was still working half the time as a judge. Now I work less, but I'm still active. I call in, and there is always a backlog, and they give me a trial. I keep up with the law, reading a daily legal newspaper, because I don't want to get on the bench and embarrass myself by not knowing about recent rulings in higher courts.

"The doctor and I have talked about keeping active in work, or some other thing that engages your mind and makes you useful. I choose to stay on the job, because without the compulsion of a job I'd tend to rot. But it doesn't have to be that. I know people who get heavily into a hobby or something like painting and that works just as well.

"My relationship with Dr. Bortz has been all about staying healthy, and that's something that has affected every aspect of my life. I feel most grateful when I'm at a school reunion, and I see classmates who were once so athletic and strong now using walkers and having trouble breathing. Or when I travel, I see people my age who can't walk 100 yards up a little hill to see a beautiful vista.

"I guess what I'm saying is that living this way, with Dr. Bortz' support, has made my life, at seventy-eight, so much more fun. Among my classmates from law school it seems like those of us who haven't had heart bypasses are a very small group. But I'm one of them and I think it's wonderful. I've outlived all the Tuttles that came before me, and I'm living pretty well, too. I couldn't ask for more."

DOCTOR

An author, public speaker, and practicing physician, Walter Bortz III was born in 1930 into a distinguished family of doctors. His father was president of the American Medical Association. His uncle Walter practiced for more than fifty years. Over the years, Bortz has moved from research on the biology of obesity to diabetes and finally geriatrics. He has also evolved into a physician-crusader for healthy living. Devoted to public health, he regards the entire American population as his community of patients. He meets many of them at public appearances such as book-signings and television tapings.

On the morning when we met at his office in the Palo Alto Health Foundation, Dr. Bortz was busy filling out an application for the Peace Corps. He explained that he had lived a very comfortable life in Palo Alto since 1972 and had decided, at age sixty-eight, that it was time to find a new challenge and a new opportunity to help others. A marathon runner, Dr. Bortz had, a day earlier, run ten miles in the nearby mountains.

"My dad was a physician who saw medicine as a calling, a true covenant, and I picked that up from him. He founded a hospital that had the promotion of health as its primary mission. He was a big believer in public health education and so am I.

"But I am more of an outlyer than he was. I see that most of medicine is doing something to the patient. It's the hospital, surgery, technology, pharmacy model. Lately it's gotten so that genes are blamed for everything. It's almost like there's been a conspiracy to promote this fatalistic notion that you can't do anything about your health. It's all predetermined. The focus is so strong that people forget that in normal people it's only a small part of their health. How we live is much more important in the long run. And I think that if we live properly, our real lifespan, the time when we can lead a high-functioning, productive life, is at least one hundred years. I think it's very exciting.

"My goal is to get Archie Bunker to realize this, to become fit, and to reach that goal. I try to do this by sharing my excitement with my patients or to people I talk to at meetings or on programs. I think we should all dare to be one hundred, and that we should realize that at that age we don't have to be very debilitated and leading a grim life. I have plenty of patients in their eighties and nineties who are doing very well.

"I am pretty sure I know what works. I communicate on a pretty intellectual basis. I appeal to people's common sense. The first thing to remember is that you either use it or you lose it. That means you have to keep moving. You have to be engaged in your life. The deterioration people see in their bodies is mostly from disuse, not age. Your diet has to be proper. You have to take responsibility for yourself. It's all pretty basic. The good news is, it's never too late to start. Some people respond to the message and do very well. None of them leave saying they didn't get the information.

"One of my more interesting patients came to me when he was sixty-three years old. He was a cardboard box manufacturer, very successful in business, but very stressed. His belly preceded him into the office. His face was red. He was pretty angry. His blood pressure and cholesterol were both high. He was a heavy smoker. I gave him a physical and noted that he was a time bomb, really. I told him what he needed to do, but I didn't see him for a year.

"When he scheduled an appointment after such a long time I was surprised that he was even still alive and able to come back. Then when he showed up, he was this slimmed-down, straight-backed fellow I almost didn't recognize. He had stopped smoking, lost fifty pounds, and was jogging five miles a day. All of this involved no medicines or technology. It didn't cost anything except his effort. But obviously he had responded very well to the information. The wonderful thing is that he realized he could do it himself, and he did.

"Many people see me very infrequently because the goal is for them to take control of their own lives. Sometimes with older people we meet more often. In any case, I'm a very low tech doctor.

"Eventually it can be almost a social thing. One woman, Florence, whom I've seen for twenty-five years, makes her visits a social outing. She has been an avid swimmer all her life and until recently lived in the same house. She's virtually blind now, which forced her into one of these apartments for assisted living. She doesn't like it much at all.

"I can see that our relationship, how I reinforce her independence and encourage her, is the most important thing. Oh, she has a little irritable bowel and some ankle swelling. If necessary I give her a little medication. But she's never in the hospital or anything like that. I respect and support her self-reliance, and I think that's the best thing I can do to keep her going.

"Checking yourself and your attitudes, is a very important part of all this. I mean, you have to know how you are coming off if you are going to relate well to people. One of the things that I have to be careful about is presenting myself as such a paragon that people decide it's unrealistic. They will say, 'I can't be like you. I can't run marathons, so forget it.'

"I remember that one time I appeared on *Sonja Live*—it's a television talk show—and I was beating my chest about all this for quite some time. I was challenging people to consider what makes a good life, to do the things that make life worthwhile.

"Well, there was this very large woman—her name was Tilly—sitting in the first row. They must have put her there on purpose. She stands up and she gives it to me. She says, 'This doctor is so pompous. When I feel like taking a walk, I lie down until it passes. If I feel like eating something, anything, I eat all that I want. I'm happy with myself, and I don't have to live like he does.'

"The audience loved her. She had deflated the arrogant doctor, put me in my place. I had let her do that because I had been too overbearing. All I could say was that as an American, I respect her right to say what she believed. But inside, I was thinking that she was being terribly self-destructive.

"When you are trying so hard to relate to people and change their behavior, you inevitably get very involved in psychology. I've seen over and over that one of the main reasons that people decline in their later years is disengagement. They withdraw from life. You see this especially with men. At sixty-five they lose their jobs. Then comes impotency. What do men care about? Sex and money. If they lose these two of major parts of their lives, it's as if they are being drummed out. Both of their epaulets are ripped off, and they feel useless. Hemingway said he could no longer write or screw. Then he killed himself.

"The problem with this, I tell men, is that if you accept this fate, then you are simply throwing away twenty, thirty or even forty years of life. But if they can make themselves healthy, and engage in something they care about, then it all comes back. It even repairs their sexuality.

"One really good example of this is a man I see who is a judge in Northern California. He is in his late seventies, and he is still active in the law. He is physically active. He pays careful attention to his diet and exercise, and he is full of energy. He is living so well because he has made himself necessary. That was my grandfather's main piece of advice to everyone. Make yourself useful.

"I tell people to think of life as a game. You get one point for a good sex life. You get one for reading, one for exercise. And you get two points for being necessary. Give yourself a score every day. The person who dies with the most points wins.

. . .

"None of what I say, about living to one hundred, or even 120, means that you don't have to deal with death. In fact, I think a lot of what I'm talking about is making your life worthwhile so that death has some dignity. I also think that understanding death improves our understanding of time. I think a lot about time and what it means to us. I think our real lifespan is about 120 years. That's one million hours. Many people have no real concept of its passage or how they are using it.

"Life does reach its end. I may say we can live to be one hundred, but the reality is most people do not, for one reason or another. That's not a failure. My experience with my patients is that most deaths are actually good. People want to die with no pain, no tubes and no loneliness, and the fact is, most do. Pain management is especially important. I give all my patients who need it morphine. There's no reason not to.

"But when it comes to other issues, like breathing tubes, everyone makes their own choices. It boils down to what that individual believes makes life valuable. For some people that means functioning very well. For others it's the ability to understand what's going on, to have memories, to squeeze a hand.

"I had a patient once who was dying of Lou Gehrig's disease. He was sixty-three. He decided he had enough. He wanted the tube out. He set up a whole schedule. His family came in to be with him. At three o'clock the tube came out. He died twenty minutes later. It was consistent with how he had lived: engaged, in control. I hope that having me as a doctor helped make that possible."

Candor, Communication,
and Concern

‽

Richard Greene, M.D., 60, dermatologist,
Plantation, Florida

Carol Rhodes, 50, designer,
Boca Raton, Florida

‽

PATIENT

Before she met Richard Greene, M.D., Carol Rhodes had already learned how to get what she needed from doctors. During
a previous health crisis she had refused to accept a dismal diagno-

sis and found a cure when she located a doctor who would listen. Years later, when she was diagnosed with cancer, she found Dr. Greene, and hope, when other doctors said there was none.

"I went to see Dr. Greene after I was diagnosed with melanoma. They thought they were just removing a cyst, but it turned out to be cancer. The first doctor I talked to said that on the scale of things, I was in the middle of the worst earthquake ever. It was like I had no chance. But when I went to the hospital for some tests, my husband sat in the waiting room with a retired radiologist who had just moved to Florida. He told us about Dr. Greene.

"The thing that impressed me from the beginning was that Dr. Greene was focused entirely on me, that he was very calm, but he was also very assertive. He was a scientific factfinder who could also be a friend. In our very first meeting he made a call to the top surgeon in our area to make sure I would be able to see him.

"Since this also started I've had several surgeries and a lot of other treatments. I have found new lumps, called him immediately, and gone in to see him right away. He doesn't make me wait and worry. He takes my fear seriously, and I appreciate that. He will call me at night at home to make sure I'm alright. And he has given me his home phone number too.

"I guess what happens when a doctor is this thorough and assertive on your behalf is that you really trust him. One example of this is that I know a lot of dermatologists keep a chart of your body and make little marks where they see something on the skin. I asked Dr. Greene why he doesn't do this. He said he knows my skin and that he checks it thoroughly every time. My level of trust is so high that I believe what he's saying, and I wouldn't ever question it again."

DOCTOR

Richard Greene realized he had a way with people when he was a seventeen-year-old in New Haven, Connecticut. His father, a real estate man, had come down with the flu on the day he was to show a Yale professor a house to buy. He asked his son to take over. When the professor balked at buying the house, Richard listened to his reasons and immediately thought of a better match. They went to see it and the professor bought it on sight.

After attending Yale University, Dr. Greene studied medicine at Harvard and did residencies in Boston area hospitals. He chose dermatology because it calls for a variety of medical skills, including surgery, and presents complex puzzles to be solved. In the time he has practiced, the rising rate of skin cancer and development of many cosmetic procedures has combined with the aging of the population to make dermatology a booming specialty. His style of relating to patients is based on three basic elements: candor, communication, and concern.

"The rate of skin cancer in Florida is probably twenty or thirty times the rate in the Northeast. There are a lot of reasons for this. One is that people do spend more time outdoors here. The other is the intensity of the sun. And you don't have to live here all your life to be at risk. A lot of older people who move here to retire have been coming to Florida every winter since they were kids. They sat out in the sun for two weeks straight every winter.

"We're not just talking about one little spot on a person's skin. It's not unusual for a patient to come in and I'll be able to see eight cancers right away, before I really examine them. I've seen as many as thirty-seven on one person. And they don't have to be old, either. One of my patients lost her son to melanoma when he was just twenty-one years old. He came in two years too late to be saved. The loss has been devastating for her. She makes appointments to come in and see me, for her own check-ups and to talk, and she cancels every one.

"The good news is that we might only have one death in a thousand skin cancer cases. But that doesn't mean that the diagnosis isn't serious, and that's probably where I start with everyone. I am always extremely honest with patients about what to expect. If a patients asks, 'I'm not going to have a scar, will I?' I know she is very concerned about it. Well, the truth is that she probably will have a scar, but we'll do our best to make it small. Or if a fifty-year-old man comes in for a hair transplant and asks, 'What will I look like?' I say, 'You're going to look like you, at fifty, but with hair.'

"The important thing is to keep the patient completely informed. I believe in full disclosure. That means telling them exactly what you are doing and explaining when you are taking the extra steps for them. People appreciate knowing you are making the effort, and it's good medicine. Try to examine all of the skin. Use magnification and lights. I also take a lot of scrapings from skin and just take them straight to the microscope. Believe it or not, a lot of doctors don't do this, even though it's often the best way to diagnose something. Patients appreciate it when you make the effort.

"It also works. I can explain how. I recently saw a lady who was itching terribly. She had been to all sorts of doctors, none of whom helped. Eventually they sent her to see a psychiatrist, who put her on Thorazine, an antipsychotic. It's true that people's psychological problems can turn up on their skin, but you have to be careful about rushing to that conclusion.

"The problem was, she was still itching. She came to see me, and I noticed that her husband was itching too. I took a scraping and ran it into a lab and found mites. She had scabies. No one had ever tried to find it. And he had it too. She didn't need Thorazine; she needed to get rid of these mites.

"Communicating very clearly with a patient and their family can make a big difference too. I took care of this ninety-nine-year-old man who had a skin cancer on his cheek. I knew about another patient, a little younger, who had come in with a similar cancer, which I didn't want to operate on because the operation was riskier than the cancer. She went to another doctor who took her into surgery. She died the next day of complications. I explained this all to the patient and the family. They were most concerned about him celebrating his one-hundredth birthday. We didn't do the surgery. It was a choice that everyone made with all the information, and I think it was the best.

"Patients are more realistic than a lot of doctors give them credit for being. An eighty-year-old woman will come into my office for laser work on her face and tell me, 'I don't have to look pretty, but I want to look better.' We can do that.

"You can show your concern for patients in a lot of ways. Touching is very important. I use my hands because I have to examine every patient's skin, but the touch also communicates caring and healing. I think it's very important.

"One technique I use is to keep cards in my pocket to make special notes. If I see a patient who needs to be followed closely I write their name and telephone number and a little note on the card. At the end of the day I call them back, just to check in. It's a good way to keep track of what's going on with them, and it's a good way to show them that you haven't forgotten about them even though you've been through a very busy day.

"I also let my patients know about me a little. I remember when my father died and I saw someone who told me she had just lost her father. We talked about that together and I think she appreciated it. I know it made me feel closer to her.

"Sometimes this can lead to some funny situations. I treat this one couple, the Steinbergs, who are very nice people. Mr. Steinberg, Sigmund, is usually very involved in life. He's very active. One time he confided in me that he was feeling depressed. He didn't know what life had left for him. I referred him to a psychiatrist and it helped.

"Anyway, I was reading the paper one morning and I saw that he had died. It had to be him. He had a very unusual name and he lived in a small town. It was all there in the paper. This was very upsetting and I called Judy, my office manager, and said we had to go to the funeral, which was that day. Fortunately

Judy went to the office and got their phone number. We called just to make sure, and there was Sig. I told him that I was getting dressed to go to his funeral, and we all laughed. But it made me realize how much I cared about him. I had been pretty upset when I read the paper. That's the risk of connecting with your patients."

Help and Self-Help

‿

Robert L. DuPont, 62, psychiatrist,
Rockville, Maryland*

"Roger," 75, businessman, Potomac, Maryland
"Anna," 46, mother, Bethesda, Maryland

‿

"ROGER," PATIENT

After building a fortune worth hundreds of millions of dollars, Roger began drinking to ease the pressures of business life. Within a few years he was beginning each day and ending each evening with alcohol. Though he believed he was unaffected by his drinking, in fact his marriage and his relationships with his sons were all damaged. In 1988, he began treatment with Dr. Robert DuPont.

"I didn't really start to drink until I was in my fifties. I really enjoyed it. I was a very busy executive. I'd get in the office at five AM and have a couple of belts right away. I'd do a little work and then have a couple more. At nine AM, when everyone came into the office, no one would think I was drunk. It was too early. But they didn't realize I had been there so long.

"Gradually it got worse. After a while I started to do things and say things that really caused problems in my family. I was obnoxious at times, but I wouldn't agree I had a problem.

"Once I had an argument with my wife. It was about midnight and I was going to meet my pilot at the airport at six AM for a trip. I packed my briefcase and said I was going to leave, do some work at the airport, and take my flight. I guess I was weaving on the highway because I got stopped. I told the police officer I didn't drink. I was just tired. But I didn't have my license on me. When I called my wife to ask her to bring it to me she said, right there on the speaker phone, 'When are you going to stop drinking?' He heard and just started laughing at me.

"Finally my sons and a friend all came to me and told me what they thought. They made it clear they believed I was an alcoholic. I agreed to see Dr. DuPont, but I still thought I was going to prove them wrong.

"Dr. DuPont was very easy to talk to. He listened very carefully. But on the second or third visit he tells me he's recommending I go to the Betty Ford clinic. He shows me this letter that he wants me to take out there with me, and he says I should read it because it's about the facts as he sees them. In the first sentence he says, 'I am sending you Roger because he is an alcoholic and a liar.'

"I was really surprised. Pretty uncomfortable with what he was saying. But I didn't argue with him. I want people to tell me what they think right out. I still didn't agree with him though. So I agreed to go to Betty Ford, but I told him they would send me back in a week with a letter saying he was wrong. I stayed for the full month. I started with Alcoholic Anonymous and I haven't had a drink in ten years. And I still see Dr. DuPont."

"ANNA," PATIENT

The child of wealthy parents, Anna was the beneficiary of a trust fund, which meant that work was not a necessity of life. However, she says of this luxury, "nothing comes for free. The trust fund is nice, but it also enabled me to get heavily into drugs." Anna was a daily cocaine abuser and had begun to dabble in heroin when she became Robert DuPont's patient. She was one of two patients who introduced him to the power of 12-step groups. She is a single parent.

"To put it bluntly, I wanted Dr. DuPont to save my life. At the time I wasn't really doing anything but using. I wasn't seeing anybody. I wasn't going out. I was just staying up days at a time. I was getting pretty paranoid, and I knew that if I didn't do something to stop I was going to die.

"I liked Dr. DuPont a lot when I first went to see him. I saw him for three or four months while I was still using cocaine. I would even use just before going to see him. He would tell me I needed to stop, and I would tell him, 'When you fix my life, then I'll be able to stop.'

"Then, all of a sudden he tells me, 'This is pointless. I can't help you unless you stop using, so why don't you just stop coming here. It's a waste of your time and money.'

"I was pretty shocked. I mean, I had gotten pretty bonded to him. This is the guy who was supposed to save my life. But then here was this ultimatum. If he wasn't going to help me, I was lost. But he was saying he was going to abandon me if I didn't stop using. He recommended I go to a twenty-four-hour treatment center and he gave me the name of this guy—Mike—who had just finished there. It turned out that I knew Mike. He had been such a mess that if treatment could help him, then I knew it could help anyone.

"Mike took me to my first Narcotics Anonymous meeting. When I got out of rehab I went to two meetings a day. Dr. DuPont wasn't sure about the whole thing. In talking to him, I could tell he didn't know much about AA or NA. But I told him that in the meetings I came to see that the whole way I was looking at life had been wrong. I was unhappy before I started using drugs. The meeting seemed to reinforce what I was realizing with Dr. DuPont, which was that I had been wrong about a lot of things.

"I had always looked to other people to make me happy, like

I was looking for him to save me. And I was always trying to control what other people were doing. Now I'm getting control of my own life, and I can see that it is the only way I'm going to have a future that is positive and safe. The other direction could kill me, literally. That's why I think treatment has saved my life."

DOCTOR

It is ironic that Dr. DuPont would become an addiction specialist, as his father was a tobacco and beer salesman. His mother went back to college in adulthood to become a teacher. When he was a boy, he lived in the Midwest, Colorado, and Atlanta. Robert's one brother also became a physician, and his one sister is a social worker.

Robert DuPont's father fought a lifelong battle with diseases real and imagined. For this reason, the DuPont family revered doctors. It was therefore no surprise that when Robert realized that he was gifted in the sciences, he chose medicine for a career. At Harvard Medical School he found psychiatry and began probing the tragic mysteries of addiction.

Between 1973 and 1978 Dr. DuPont was the director of the National Institute on Drug Abuse and "drug czar" leading the White House's campaign against drug abuse. It wasn't until he entered full-time medicine as a psychiatrist that he discovered, with the help of his patients, the ideas that are now the foundation of his practice. The cornerstone is self-help, in the style of Alcoholics Anonymous, which he says is the "secret weapon" in the war against drugs.

. . .

"One day when I was a kid, my father just announced we were moving to Denver. It was for his health. Some doctor told him it would be good for his asthma, and so he did it. That's the way he was.

"For the first four months we lived in a motel. The only thing there was around there was a library. I went all the time. I remember I found this big black book, *The Human Mind,* by Karl Menninger. It really excited me. He had all these ways to fix people. Even then I think I was looking for answers, maybe trying to fix my father, who really was a hypochondriac.

"From the very beginning, from my first exposure to psychiatry in medical school, I was deeply interested in the stories of my patients. In psychiatry words, feelings, and relationships are everything. Some therapists believe that the patient comes into treatment already knowing everything and that you just have to help them get it out. That's not entirely crazy. But I think there should be more of a relationship. People come to me because I've seen a lot of people who have had similar problems. I'm not going to withhold what I know.

"Patients also come to me with their own insights. I learned about 12-step groups from two patients—both middle-class heroin addicts—who literally turned their lives around in Narcotics Anonymous. One was a terrible drug addict who managed to recover. He told me the difference between himself and his peers was the 12 steps. He was a very insightful guy. I didn't know anything about the program and he taught me a lot.

"The other patient was this woman who was his friend. He introduced her to Narcotics Anonymous and it worked for her too. They went to these meetings every day in the beginning, and they would tell me about them. You couldn't help seeing that it helped. When they stayed with the program, they were able to stop using the drugs. When they stopped going, they relapsed. One of these patients was sober for seventeen years. She stopped going, thought she was done. Then she relapsed after seventeen years of not using.

"The amazing thing to me today is I can still go to meetings of doctors, and they are ignorant about 12-step programs. Most doctors still don't know much about them, and they are not really receptive to the idea that they might work. Of course, at the same time most doctors really don't want to treat addicts. They think it's hopeless. I've come to believe that the major thing in addiction treatment is education and plugging a patient into Alcoholics Anonymous or Narcotics Anonymous.

"There are exceptions, but only a few. I have one patient who's a very high-powered computer genius. He's had a drug problem since college. I insisted that he go to 12-step meetings but he refused. He has stopped using drugs, and I don't think he'll have a relapse. The reason? Stubbornness. He wants to show me that he doesn't need it. That's part of the relationship. In this case, it's working.

"The relationship between the therapist and the patient is the heart of psychiatry. I won't just prescribe pills for someone and let them go. Psychotherapy has to be part of the treatment. Over the years, I've refined the way I think about this relationship. People have this phrase 'using a doctor.' It used to be that I didn't like that expression. But I do now. I want to be used. I consider myself as the agent of the patient. I am there quite literally to be used by them.

"One part of that is getting them to the point where they take full responsibility for their addiction. It's one of the twelve steps and it's absolutely critical. People will blame everything and every one, but my experience is that people stay sick until they look at themselves. I'm into honesty. I'm honest with my patients, and I try to help them to be honest with themselves.

"Often that doesn't happen to an addict until they hit bottom. That can be very frightening. My cousin Donny, a cocaine and alcohol addict, sat down next to me at a family reunion a while back. He had already been arrested for selling drugs. Anyway, he sat down next to me and put a beer in front of himself. I know exactly what he's saying with that, and so does he. He says to me, 'Bob, I haven't had enough.' Six months later, at three AM, he finally had enough. He was killed in a car crash. That was how he hit bottom.

"But in most cases, it doesn't have to go that far. If you build some trust, you can be very blunt with people and it works. I had this sixty-five-year-old patient who was one of the most successful executives in America, and an alcoholic. He didn't want to see it. I told him what I saw, that he was an alcoholic and a liar. I recommended he go to Betty Ford. This man looked at my recommendation as a challenge. He hasn't had a drink in ten years. That's pretty rewarding for him and for me. That's what being honest and taking responsibility can do."

Hometown Hero

❧

Helen Cappuccino, M.D., 35, general surgeon,
Lockport, New York

Ross Lown, 69, retired salesman,
Lockport, New York

❧

PATIENT

Ross Lown was first diagnosed with emphysema in 1985. A salesman by trade, he found it increasingly difficult to make his rounds.
He first met Dr. Cappuccino in 1994 when she performed a

bronchoscopy on him. He would not become her regular patient until one year later, when he turned to her during a crisis.

"I remember in 1994 I was in the hospital throwing up blood and they brought this little lady in to do a bronchoscopy. This young little woman comes in and stands by my bed. The first thing I thought was, give her a quarter and tell her to come back when she graduates. When she told me her name, I immediately had a joke for her. 'Oscar Meyer has a hot dog truck,' I said. 'What do you drive, a cup or a mug?' She gave me this big smile and I knew it was going to be alright. One of the strongest medicines is a sense of humor and she obviously has one. I let her have it and she did a good job.

"Then in 1995 I got really bad. I was having a lot of trouble breathing. A pretty big part of my lung had stopped functioning and was pressing on my heart. My family physicians told me there was nothing more they could do for me. I remember I was in the hospital. I told them that I was just going to get a bottle of wine and a bottle of sleeping pills, and go home and die.

"That day Dr. Cappuccino came in the room to see the patient next to me. I told her what was happening and I asked her to operate on me. There's a way they can take out the bad part of the lung and it can help. But it's risky and at first she told me it wasn't possible, my body couldn't take it. But she said she would think about it.

"Well, I think she talked to my other doctors and heard what I had said because the next day she came in and told me to make an appointment at her office for as soon as I got out. They would do some tests on me, and if I passed, she would try to operate.

The tests showed my heart was fine, but I had trouble getting up to the level they wanted on the breathing. I was down to ninety-three pounds and pretty weak. The thing was, I got better each time they tried it, so eventually they said, 'It looks like he's got the will to make himself do it.'

"I think you've got to understand what a risk Dr. Cappuccino took and why I trusted her. I only had a 10 percent chance of surviving and even then it wasn't for sure that I would be able to breathe any better. But she is probably the most intelligent person I ever met. The minute she opens her mouth, her intelligence snaps you to attention. She's also one of the most caring people I know. She knew I wanted to try this, and that I was willing to risk it. I told her she should do her best and whatever happens, it's alright with me. We were in it together.

"The day of the operation she shows up in the morning and I have a little fun with her. It was the day the jury gave the verdict in the O.J. Simpson case, and I told her I wanted to delay until I heard it. She laughed and we went ahead with the operation. The next thing I know I'm hearing people shouting two things at me: 'Ross, wake up,' and 'O.J. Simpson's not guilty.'

"I did much better after that operation. Because she took a chance on me, I've had three good years I never expected to have. We are very lucky here in Lockport to have someone as capable as her. And needless to say, I'm in love with her."

DOCTOR

"There's a saying about surgery. 'Either you cure them or you kill them.' That's not exactly true, but it's sort of close. That's why I like it, actually. There's a lot of satisfaction, a lot of gratification that comes from performing an operation when it goes well.

"When it does go well, I am bound to run into a patient later because this is a very small town, actually. I'll either see them at the supermarket or they'll pop into the office, and it is always nice. I've seen them through something traumatic, something they were fearful about, and it came out okay. There's a bond between us and I don't try to deny that.

"I don't deny it when it doesn't work out, either. That's why I go to funerals. A lot of doctors say I shouldn't do that, but I disagree. I knew that person, and I was involved with them during a very important time in their life. I think it's appropriate to go, and I think families appreciate it. I get some closure out of it too. It's not just for them.

"But this is getting ahead of things. You start the relationship with the patient by asking a lot of questions about their lives. If they've been referred to you for vague abdominal pain—and I get a lot of referrals like that—then I ask about the things that are obviously stressful in life. There's often something about marriage or kids and that's what's causing the pain. It's real pain, but it won't be helped by surgery.

"You don't get to this kind of stuff if you don't talk with your patients. But you also have to be prepared for what comes out when you do. I once had a patient come in to have a repair done on a hernia operation. She hadn't followed the instructions for rest after the first operation, and we went over them in detail. Eventually it came out that she couldn't comply the first time because she's in a very abusive marriage, and her husband didn't allow her to take the time off she needed.

"What was interesting was that she had put up with abuse for years, but hearing from me that it was wrong really made an impression. I liked her, and it disturbed me to hear that this was going on. We continued to talk about it during follow-up visits. I referred her to a support group and, wouldn't you know it, she got out of that relationship. It all started with her having someone listen and validate her sense that what was going on was wrong.

"I want people to know that I am there to use my skills in the way they want, and that I will do it if it can possibly help them. Maybe the best example is a man who had lung disease and was so disabled by it that he really couldn't move five feet without losing his breath and needing to sit down.

"Now, technically, his lung capacity was already reduced to the point where it was supposedly incompatible with life. But the body adjusts to that, and he was living, but in a very compromised way. It is possible in such cases to remove a portion of the lung that is not functioning and actually improve things, at least temporarily. But it can be a controversial thing to do. The mortality rate is high, and there's a possibility that the patient would require a ventilator for the rest of their life.

"In this case the patient really wanted to go through with it. He made it clear to me that he didn't want to go on with life as it was. He was a very nice man, very sweet. He said, 'I'd rather die in the hands of a beautiful woman like you than go on like this. It's my choice to do it.'

"If there was absolutely no chance that it would help, and it was certain he would die because of the operation, then I would refuse to do it. But that wasn't the case. There was a chance it would relieve his suffering. And I feel that I have this certain skill that ethically I'm obliged to make available for people if they want it. This case worked out very well. He had a good recovery and his symptoms were relieved. We were both glad we did it.

"In other cases the relationship is a little less balanced. This is when patients need me to be more of an authority figure, like a parent. The irony is that I am practicing in a town where I was a little girl. There are people I put pacemakers into who gave me lollipops when I was little. Others I have to read the riot act to, so they will keep up with their medication or take symptoms seriously.

"A lot of people in town know quite a bit about me. My father is a dentist here, my mother a lawyer. It's a pretty prominent family, and when I got pregnant at seventeen and had a baby, people knew about that, too. But what's interesting is that no one judges me negatively for that. They sort of see it as a glitch, the kind of thing that happens to teenagers, and they respect me for still going on with life, and for coming back to Lockport to live and practice medicine. This history I think gives me a connection to people.

"I also feel like I have a personality that allows me to win a patient's trust. This helps especially when the news is bad, someone's dying, and you have to help break the denial in a family. People have to believe that you will always tell them the truth and that you have their best interest at heart. I do.

"I also get something back, and that's what makes practicing in a small town where you grew up special. My patients know me. The last time I had a baby I received little booties patients had knitted and baby clothes. I run into people at the supermarket and we talk about our lives. That's the wonderful part about it all. No matter how brief the contact may be, my relationships are meaningful. I make a mark. I affect their lives, and that makes me feel good."

PART THREE

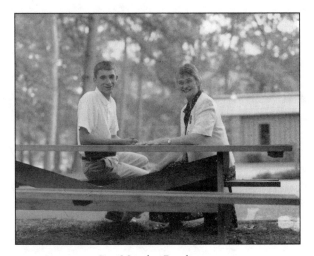

Dr. Marsha Raulerson

The

Mentors

Physician as Mentor

∽

Greta Rainsford, M.D., 61, pediatrician,
Hempstead, New York

Tondawa Coles, M.D., 26, pediatrician,
Philadelphia, Pennsylvania

∽

PATIENT

Tondawa Coles was five years old when she became Dr. Rainsford's patient. Already diagnosed with sickle cell anemia, Towanda spent far more time with Dr. Rainsford than a typical patient.

At the age of twenty-six, Tondawa became Dr. Coles and began a three-year residency in pediatrics at Albert Einstein Hospital in Philadelphia.

"Actually, Dr. Rainsford reminded me of my Dad. She was both strict and kind. You could tell she was serious about what she was doing, but that made me feel confident, like everything was going to be alright.

"She was strict, because I think she felt that a lot of the families she dealt with needed that. But she also listened. I remember once when I was in the hospital and Christmas was coming. I wasn't all better. I had fever and pain. And she thought I should stay. I know I started to cry. When she saw how upset I was about not going home, she agreed to release me. My mother got a lot of instructions about what to do, and she checked on me a lot. But I think I recovered better at home than I would have at the hospital because I was so much happier.

"Dr. Rainsford had a good relationship with my mother. I remember they would talk a long time, and sometimes really laugh together. Dr. Rainsford knew my family well.

"When I was young, it didn't seem unusual to me to have a black woman who was my doctor. But as I got older I realized how special it was. She became my role model. In high school there was a teacher who told me I just wasn't cut out to be a doctor, that I couldn't handle it, even though I was getting the highest grades. The same thing happened in college, when my mentor said I was making a mistake. I thought of what Dr. Rainsford would do. I got another mentor.

"In medical school they have tried to teach us about establishing a good rapport with patients, but that's not something you can really pick up from a lecture. I think it comes over time. I've been influenced more by the fact that I was a patient so much as a child, and by Dr. Rainsford.

"In the pediatrics clinic I see patients on a regular basis. A lot of them come from poorer parts of the inner city where there are a lot of social problems and parents who are under a lot of stress. I spend a little more time with them, and I try to be in tune with their emotional side. I watch the interactions of parents and children, and I will say something to a mother if something doesn't look right. I am careful not to alienate her. I want her to know I'm on her side. But I guess, like Dr. Rainsford, I think it's my responsibility, because the child is the patient, to speak up when I should."

DOCTOR

Though she was a little girl at the time, Greta Rainsford knew that a chance encounter with a doctor who was both African-American and female was a fleeting glimpse of her future. In the late 1940s African-American women doctors were rare, even in Harlem. When high-school teachers suggested secretarial training, she demanded college. Medical school followed.

Now in her early sixties, Greta Rainsford, M.D., is the pediatrician for two thousand children in the lower-middle income New York suburb of Hempstead.

. . .

"In pediatrics, the child is your patient. I came out of my training with that idea, and I have never had trouble relating to the babies and children. I hold babies, and take my time to make sure they feel safe. As the children get older, I help them become more involved in their own care. When a child is fourteen, I usually kick the parent out. It's part of their development to learn how to take care of themselves, and they need some privacy. What they tell me is confidential, unless there's an absolute need for parents to know.

"At first, I had trouble with the parents. I admit, I didn't like them that much. They often didn't follow my instructions, or they would do things that would make a situation worse. But I needed the parents as my collaborators in treating the child.

"When you get to know the family, especially those who are poor, you realize that there's a complex environment that child lives in. I found I was treating children for allergies or something similar, and they weren't getting better. If I paid a visit to the house, I could get a much better idea of the foods the family was eating and the dust problems in the house. I believe in fresh air. Lower the thermostat. Open the window. Put on a sweater if you are cold. When you visit someone's house, you can go over all of this right there.

"The child also has parents and other children and grandparents. Often you'll tell a parent to do something with a baby. They go home and the grandmother will tell them to do the opposite. Also, there are parents who can't read. Or they don't understand English well enough to follow what you are saying. They nod. I ask them if they have any questions, and they say, 'No.' I then give them written materials and go over it again, just in case.

"When I went to medical school, they didn't teach us anything about relating to parents. They didn't tell me that parents are anxious and sometimes pretty crazy acting. Some parents don't even know how to feed their baby, to stop when the baby stops moving his mouth. When they have older children they don't know how to set limits. Talking about all of this is part of the relationship.

"I was doing managed care long before people were really using that term. I would tell parents to stay out of the emergency room for routine problems. I am available twenty-four hours a day, seven days a week. I want the child to see me for continuity of care, not a doctor that they'll probably never see again.

"One good way to explain why this is is to look at the abuse of antibiotics. Emergency rooms diagnose a lot of otitis media and give out a lot of antibiotics when I don't see anything in the ear or it's obviously something viral. That's how we've gotten these bugs that are so resistant to the drugs. I spend a lot of time training my patients' parents to understand that they don't need to leave the office with a prescription every time. But if they go to the emergency room, it's automatic. That's lousy care.

"There's also a lot of ways you have to help parents so that their child grows up strong mentally and emotionally. That's important because if your head is screwed up, your body gets screwed up too. I tell parents that they are the small society where the child is going to learn about how life works. The real society isn't going to be as kind or pleasant as they are. So I encourage them to create structure, establish consequences for a child's actions, and stick by them. There is no physical violence. I won't tolerate that. But when they say something, they have to mean it, so a child feels secure, because there are boundaries and he or she learns there are consequences in this world.

"I am just as direct with parents. I guide with authority. I tell them that if they want me to be their child's doctor, they have to cooperate. They have to trust me and follow my directions when their child is sick. They see that it works, that what I'm asking them to do turns out better than what grandma is telling them. They have to say, 'Grandma, you raised your babies. Now you let me raise mine.'

"When the child becomes fourteen, I want to see them on their own. The goal is to foster independence and a sense of responsibility in the child. I also want them to feel there is someone they can go to. I've been able to help girls with pregnancies who were afraid to tell their parents, because they literally believed their fathers might kill them. I've also identified situations where the mother is subtly encouraging adolescent daughters to have babies. The families are poor. The mothers had babies when they were very young, and deep down they want to have another baby in the house. I spend a lot of time talking to these girls. I help them to resist being manipulated.

"The idea of women being strong in the family, of getting respect, and being the real link between people is a part of the African-American culture. It doesn't come from Africa so much as it comes from our experience here. It started with slavery. Slavery broke up families, but mainly it separated men from their wives and children. Mothers became the heads of families.

"Today, the obstacles that young Black men face are probably the greatest that anyone has to deal with. That's one reason why there are so many female-headed families. What it all means, though, is people are used to taking women, especially older Black women, seriously. There is more of a matriarchy. It doesn't always work in my favor. I've encountered some men, some fathers, who really can't deal with me. But mostly the people in my practice are willing to depend on me. They want me to be the source of information and guidance that will help them.

"I do establish a bond with families and children. I've made an arrangement with my insurance carrier so that I can see a few adults, because some of these patients don't want to let go. They get into their twenties, but still they want to see me. I go to their weddings and take care of their children. Some of them have also become doctors. One is a young Black woman who was a foster child. She told me she was going to be a doctor, and I could see, even when she was a child, that she was going to do it. Maybe our relationship had something to do with what she's been able to accomplish. I hope so."

The Family
Medical Expert

❧

Theodore E. Wymslo, M.D., 46, general practice,
Dayton, Ohio

Rev. Roger Coulbertson, 63, pastor,
Defiance, Ohio

❧

PATIENT

Rev. Coulbertson was attending a church convention in Dayton when he suddenly felt pressure and pain in his arm and neck. Coulbertson knew all the warning signs of a heart attack.

Geraldine, his wife of forty-two years, and his two sons-in-law who are also pastors, took him to the nearest hospital, Miami Valley Hospital, an eight-hundred-bed tertiary-care center where Dr. Theodore Wymslo was on call. Their relationship would last a few short days, but leave a lasting impression.

"Looking back at it, I'd say that Dr. Wymslo was at a disadvantage because he didn't know that he was dealing with one of the angriest men in the world, but that's what I was when he came to see me. I had been in the emergency room for four hours and nothing had been done. They had lost my EKG report. I was feeling like I was in one of those gas stations where they tell you that you need a new fan belt and then put some shoe polish on the one you've got. For all I knew, they just wanted another eighty dollars for another EKG.

"I wanted to delay having any procedures done. For one thing, I was far away from home. There were no hotel rooms in the whole city for my family because the ham radio operators were having their convention in Dayton. And another thing was that the first doctors said it looked like I didn't have a heart attack. Now Dr. Wymslo comes in and says I might need angioplasty. I felt like he was slipping into his 'The Doctor is God' attitude. Doctors aren't accustomed to people questioning them. I was questioning everything."

Rev. Coulbertson explained to Dr. Wymslo that he didn't have that much faith in this procedure because of the experience of one of his colleagues. "I know the district superintendent for the Assembly of God has had eleven different things done—angioplasty and bypasses—and he's no better than when he started. Then I said something that I know got to him. I said, 'You make mistakes, doctor, and I know because I'm the one who buries your mistakes.' He couldn't have liked that one bit."

After much discussion, Rev. Coulbertson agreed to stay the night, but warned that he planned to leave at dawn. In the morning, tests showed elevated levels of enzymes that indicated a more serious heart condition. Rev. Coulbertson recalls that it was ten AM, and he was already feeling impatient when Dr. Wymslo returned to resume the debate over his immediate future.

"When he told me I should stay, I went pretty heavy on him. I said, 'Now look, I've just about had it with you and this hospital. This is more like a band-aid station than anything else. You're dealing with one of the most angry people you'll ever meet, and I want to get out of here.'

"It was about this time that I found out that if I did sign myself out my insurance company wouldn't pay the bill. The ambulance home was going to cost us another one thousand, five hundred dollars at least. And then the hospital told us they had old dorm rooms they could let my family have for twenty dollars a piece. That was within what was in our wallets. And I also found out [my insurance company] is one of the preferred providers for cardiac centers. I realized that God must have put me in this place for a reason, so I accepted it."

During the cardiac catheterization, doctors in Dayton found substantial blockage in three of Rev. Coulbertson's coronary arteries. Stints were installed and Rev. Coulbertson's recovery was quick. Five weeks later, he was up and about, building a concrete ramp for a small outbuilding at his church.

"When I cooled off, I knew that Dr. Wymslo was only concerned about my health. He was only thinking about what was best for me. But he didn't know that I've seen a lot of people die in my forty-two years as a pastor. I've been in a lot of rooms with people who are having angioplasty. My father died when he was fifty-one. My grandfather at fifty-six. My idea was to delay having anything at all done for as long as possible until I couldn't avoid it. I guess I happened to reach that point in Dayton. If I hadn't had the fear of God put into me, I wouldn't have been in that hospital at all.

"I guess my attitude was a big problem. He had to deal with a sixty-three-year-old, gray-haired man who acts like he knows it all. And I'm telling him that if they make a mistake with me it's going to be ashes to ashes, dust to dust.

"I guess I admire Dr. Wymslo for how he handled it. I'm having a fight with my doctor at home now over all this rehab stuff. I don't see why I have to go. I have my own blood pressure cuff. If they gave me an EKG machine and taught me how to read it I could take care of myself. Here I am carrying eighty-pound bags of concrete and I have a nurse telling me that I shouldn't carry more than ten pounds in each hand. I had to say what I thought of that. Of course, I know I'm not right about everything. But I have my own ideas. It's the way I am."

DOCTOR

Theodore Wymslo, son of a band-leader-turned-salesman and a homemaker mother, grew up poor in Toledo, Ohio in the 1950s and '60s. The middle child of six, he learned to love gardening by working in the plots that helped to feed his family. The aptitude test he took in high school showed he would be a fine farmer. But a menial job inside the forensic ward at a psychiatric hospital gave him the chance to see doctors working with patients—some in leg irons—whose conditions actually improved. He decided then and there to tend to people instead of plants.

Dr. Wymslo, who turned forty-six in 1998, learned medicine at Ohio State University. But he began his lifelong education in the doctor-patient relationship during a residency at a country doctor's office in London, Ohio. Over the years he has cultivated an idiosyncratic approach to this partnership of healing. He follows each patient's lead, trying always to understand them in the context of a full life led outside whatever disease or medical crisis is at hand. He also relies on family and friends, and especially on the person he calls "the family medical expert."

"I saw the kind of doctor I wanted to be in a rural medical practice where I did a residency. The first thing I learned was that the patients often have tremendous insight into what's wrong. And a lot of the time they will tell you exactly what it is, if they trust you and believe in you.

"Back then I would have a patient and immediately start chasing every somatic complaint: headaches, stomachaches, fatigue. That's the most difficult thing doctors do, chasing these vague complaints. Then the older doctor would come in and sit down at eye level with them and wait until they got really focused on their problem. It was obvious that the patients were waiting to be certain that the doctor really cared about them. They were testing him. When they got their answer, when they saw he was really listening, they opened up. People know their bodies. They'll tell you what's wrong if you are willing to listen.

"Families test you, too. They want to see if you respect them. Most families have what I call the family medical expert. Usually, it's a woman. Sometimes this person has some medical background. Maybe they work in a hospital, or are a nurse. Sometimes it's a doctor.

"Most doctors really don't want to get involved with this person because it's a threat. In fact, in medical school we were taught to do our rounds before seven o'clock because otherwise we might bump into a patient's family. I can understand that. I mean, you are the one with a medical degree, but the patient is more interested in what their aunt has to say. If, as a doctor, you don't have that person on your side, then things are going to be a lot more difficult. So I always want to know who the family medical expert is and then I want to talk to them.

"On a practical level it usually works this way: Say a new mother wants to talk about introducing solid foods. That's a variable thing and families have strong beliefs. I ask her who she goes to for advice. If it's her own mother or grandmother, then I ask her to bring that person next time she comes in. The family medical expert is usually pleased to be involved. We'll talk and if

I disagree I'll explain why, even share some of the literature. We almost always come up with something that's acceptable to everyone.

"Of course, sometimes it's something that's much more dramatic. A few years ago I had an Asian man come in with what was assumed to be pneumonia. He had lost a lot of weight. It was possible that there was a cancer that was causing fluid to build up. He was in his fifties. He had sepsis, but he was competent mentally. I was going to tell him that he might have this cancer and that once he was treated for the pneumonia and recovered, he could go through some tests and then maybe surgery and other therapies.

"In this family the medical expert was his sister. When I told the family what I thought was going on they insisted that I not tell him. The whole family was adamant about it. 'You can't tell him he has cancer,' they said. 'That is what will kill him.'

"I talked with the sister and she explained that in their culture you don't tell someone they have cancer because they give up. The family was his support system, and they were telling me how he would respond. They were asking me to understand this as a doctor. I had to believe them. But I also needed some way that I could talk to him about the tests that he would need down the road. The sister agreed that if he got well enough to have the tests, I could come to her and we would work together.

"In the end, he didn't ever recover. He got worse, went unconscious and died of an overwhelming infection. But the family's experience made them trust Western medicine a lot more. They became regular patients in our practice and we were able to give them all care they would have otherwise resisted.

.   .   .

"It's much more common of course to have patients who present a lot of vague complaints. It can be very frustrating. Everybody calls them a 'difficult patient.' This is the person with a hundred-and-one complaints, none of which are very significant or specific. They have a stomachache, a headache, sometimes there's joint pain and fatigue. They show up with long lists. The obsessive-compulsive ones have them organized into organ systems.

"When they first see you in the office they build you up. 'We've heard you are a very caring physician, that you are very, very good.' Then out comes the list. They've gone on the Internet or to the library. They've done their research and they have a lot to say. Now they want to see how you react. Will you respect them? They are sizing you up.

"Well, the truth is, I like the ones who have their lists and research and are very organized because it helps me. And I have also learned to take these patients seriously because there have been times when I've been covering for a doctor and diagnosed a late-stage cancer in a patient who they had seen recently. It's quite possible they missed it because they were tired of listening to a difficult patient.

"Of course this doesn't mean I have the time to hear every last detail of every symptom. Recently I had a couple in their sixties come in. They both had lists with more than a hundred things on them. I explained that I didn't want to rob the next patient of their time, but that I would schedule an appointment when I can go over everything. Then I asked them to tell me their number-one priority. I told them to pick out the most important thing. We dealt with that, and then I told them we would go over the rest over a number of visits. It worked. And you do it because even though 99 percent of headaches are nothing serious, you never know if that other one percent is sitting right in front of you.

"Sometimes, especially when you are on call in the hospital, you don't have a lot of follow-up visits to work through a patient's problems and you don't have an ally in the family either. Sometimes you just come into a situation that's a crisis. Everyone's excited. Maybe the patient is mad as hell. Maybe the nurses are upset. Anyone can make a situation like this worse. The big challenge is to make it better.

"Recently I was working in the hospital when this man in his sixties came in with chest pain. He was a church pastor from—and this is perfect—a town in northern Ohio called Defiance. He was mad as hell. He starts telling me all the things that have gone wrong. He had to wait thirty minutes for pain medication. The patient across the hall has been disturbing him. 'This is a band-aid station,' he says. 'I want to be transferred to the Medical College of Ohio in Toledo. That's the best hospital in the state and I want to go there.'

"Now the nurses are very upset and so is the resident. He wants me to lay down the law with these people, be the authority, argue with them if we have to.

"But I can see that I don't have any allies in the family. His son-in-law and wife are with the patient but this is a very powerful personality—some small-town pastors get very used to having it go their way—and he's obviously in charge. They are going to do exactly what he wants and he wants to leave. I really don't have any option—he's not giving anyone any option—except to give him what he wants. So I say, 'Okay, great. If I can transport you I will.' Now the resident is glaring at me, and so are the nurses. But they don't say anything. They are waiting to see how it works out.

"Now I tell the patient that his job is to rest and relax. I ask his wife to call her insurance company and find out which hospitals they have as preferred providers for cardiac care. I ask the son-in-law to look into arranging transportation by ambulance. He comes back and says that the ambulance is four hundred dollars plus four dollars per mile. That's about one thousand dollars to get him to Toledo, and it's not covered. Then the wife comes back and she says that the hospital in Toledo is not on the insurance company's provider list. They've told her that Toledo's outcome data for heart patients is not as good as ours, and that we are one of three heart centers they cover 100 percent.

"It doesn't take very long for the pastor to decide he's going to stay right where he is. I recommend a cardiologist who I know grew up on a farm in Northern Ohio, pretty close to Defiance. He had angioplasty and the last I heard he's doing pretty well. That was the outcome we were going for. I just didn't force it to happen my way."

Ultimately, a physician who listens to his patients will have to accept even their decision to stop treatment and submit to medicine's archenemy, death. Dr. Wymslo says that this, too, is more readily done when the doctor views a patient in the context of the patient's full life, rather than the limited circumstances faced during an illness.

"One of my patients is an older woman who has already dealt with cancer before. She's got heart problems and now some masses have shown up in her lungs. It's cancer and she could undergo treatment. But the treatment is severe, and given her heart condition it could push her over the edge. She told me, 'I'd prefer to not do it.'

"Now is that a reasonable decision? How should I respond? Well, I know that she has a good relationship with her daughter and support in the community. I also know she has very strong faith. She believes in God. She's led a very, very good life and she feels it's alright for her to move to heaven.

"I didn't argue it with her. She has her own beliefs and I support people in their beliefs. Was she making a reasonable choice? After listening to her, I could see she was completely rational. She wasn't suicidal or even depressed. It was her choice. I helped make it possible for her to make it."

Doctor Mom

Marsha Raulerson, M.D., 48, pediatrician and
family physician, Brewton, Alabama

The children of Ruby McCurdy, 33, nurse,
Brewton, Alabama

PATIENT

Ruby McCurdy was born in the same small hospital in Brewton where she now works as a nurse. She first met Dr. Raulerson when she was sixteen, shortly after the birth of her first child,

Kenneth, who is now seventeen. Dr. Raulerson has also cared for her daughter, Ashley, twelve, and son, Allen, nine.

"Dr. Raulerson hadn't been practicing for very long when we first went to see her. I was sixteen and I had just had Kenny. He was two weeks old. My momma went with me, because I was so young and because she was the kind of person who just had to be involved.

"The thing I remember most about that time was that my momma and Dr. Raulerson had very strong feelings about whatever came up. My momma had raised six children, and she was sure she knew it all. Dr. Raulerson was very smart, and she had studied everything there is to know about what was right for children, and she didn't hold anything back.

"That first time, the issue was pacifiers. My mother did not believe in the pacifier at all. She never let her children have them, and she didn't think I should do it either. But Dr. Raulerson thinks that a pacifier can soothe a baby, that it can help strengthen the baby's gums, and that they don't cause the harm folks used to think they caused.

"The important thing about this is not what I decided. I was sixteen at the time, and I had just had a baby. I wasn't going to do anything against my mother. But [Dr. Raulerson] made sure to tell me that the choice was mine. She made me start thinking that I was the mother of this child and that what I felt mattered. She made me feel like my instincts were good. She said, 'This is your baby, you do what you think is right.' I was raised in a family that did not give me that kind of encouragement. She supported me. I liked that. I've also tried to do the same with my children. I encourage them the way that Dr. Raulerson does.

"In a way, Dr. Raulerson is like a mother to the mothers who bring her their children. She cares about me and how I'm doing, and she respects me. But she also has very strong ideas, and a lot of people can't appreciate that. I know there are nurses in the nursery who think that she goes overboard with her babies, asking them to do too much. But that's just because Dr. Raulerson cares, and she thinks all babies deserve the best, no matter what.

"Take education. I was raised out in the country. We had horses and cows and chickens, and doing your chores was more important than getting good grades in school. With my children it has been the opposite. I really encourage them to do their best in school. I'm not really hard on them. But if I think they could do better, I let them know that I don't think they are working up to their potential.

"This was also something I learned from Dr. Raulerson, but in a different way. She was one of the people who really encouraged me and inspired me to go back to school for nursing. When I finished, she told me about a job in the hospital nursery and I got it. Now I'm taking my first class towards becoming an RN. I think Dr. Raulerson really helped me get motivated to do this, and I think it's been good for my children to see their mother taking her own education seriously.

"Of course, Dr. Raulerson is not just someone who encourages people. She is a very good, very fine doctor. My children have been very healthy, but you can still see she's good with them. She lets them do the talking as much as possible and she treats them with respect.

"I've seen more how she handles problems when she's with other patients, like at the hospital. Once there was a mother who came in with a child—a sixth-month-old—with a big cyst at the bottom of her spine. It had obviously been there for a long while and the mother had ignored it. It was interfering with the baby's movement and would make it hard for her to sit up and crawl.

"Well, Dr. Raulerson wouldn't let that mother leave until she had called to Birmingham, found a surgeon to take care of this, and made an appointment for the mother to go there. She even found a program that would cover all of the cost, so the mother couldn't say she hadn't done it because she was too poor. She wasn't going to let that child or that mother out of her sight until she was sure the right thing was being done.

"The same thing happens in the hospital nursery. When we have a problem and we contact other doctors about what we should do, they often say, 'Well, what would Dr. Raulerson do?' Other times when we have a baby in there and we can't get the doctor to come in, we'll call Dr. Raulerson at home. She'll come see that baby, whether it's her patient or not, and whether she's on call or not. That's just the way she is. She's strong. She speaks her mind. But it's all for the children. I wouldn't have it any other way for my children's doctor.'"

DOCTOR

When her husband, Daniel, a doctor, was sent to serve in Vietnam, Marsha Raulerson began reading the copies of the *New England Journal of Medicine* that were delivered to her home. A school teacher, she was working on a doctorate in education. But as she learned about medicine, she began to feel a calling, like a religious calling, to pediatrics. She went to medical school at the University of Florida and served residencies in Pensacola.

Brewton, Alabama, is so small that its telephone listings take up just twenty-five pages in the regional directory. Forty-eight-year-old Dr. Raulerson is one of just half a dozen doctors in town. She oversees residents in pediatrics, who rotate through her office on an annual basis. Most choose to live in an apartment she has set up in her own home. Raulerson says that her practice, which requires her to be on call most of the time, is an expression of her religious faith.

"Probably one of the most important things to keep in mind, as you are trying to establish a relationship, is that there is no typical patient, no typical mother and child. I had my first child when I was twenty-nine years old and I was so excited. I became a doctor later in life, and the truth is, I didn't comprehend that there were people in this world who had babies without really wanting them. But that does happen here. We have a lot of young, poor mothers who don't plan to have children, they just do.

"This problem was discussed at a conference I went to in Tuscaloosa about eight years ago. The question was, 'What are we going to do about all these young single mothers having babies?' I think that to some degree it comes from the fact that these young women do not feel a sense of worth in their own lives. They were not loved, cherished, and wanted as newborns. We have to make sure that they do that for their own children, so that maybe they'll grow up with more of a sense of self and a sense of purpose.

"I'm working with a mother in that situation right now. She's just delivered twins. She doesn't seem to be showing much interest. In fact, her mother is more involved than she is. I know that we definitely have to encourage her to hold the babies, connect with them. We also will make sure that she's enrolled in Partners for Tomorrow. It's a program we have that sends neighbors to homes to visit with new Moms. They do pretty much what I do. They don't tell the Moms to do this and do that. They just visit and model appropriate behavior with the baby. They pick up the baby and talk to her directly. The mothers see this, and when the visitor leaves, they do it too.

"On the other hand, some very young mothers are very astute, while older ones who you think should be experienced have problems. And there's no guarantee that even if there is an extended family around that it is going to help.

"I'll give you an example. I have this family I take care of, and the mother's name is Ruby. She was a teenage mother. Her mother-in-law didn't approve of her at all, and I could see that it was making her self-conscious. She doubted herself. So I found myself giving her reinforcement for her own choices. I supported her decisions, helped her to feel more confident about her own abilities. It was as if I balanced out the mother-in-law. That was important. I think it was the best thing I could do for her as a parent.

"You figure out how to approach families based on the context of their lives. I'm not talking about their medical history. It's how they live. I used to be much tougher about things, before I understood what the context meant.

"I have this family that's headed by a man who's in his thirties, his hair is down his back and is always dirty from head to toe. His work is in a junkyard. He married this seventeen-year-old, and they started having children.

"They loved their children very much. Both of them came to the appointments, but one of the main problems was hygiene. I had to teach them about cleanliness. At one point they told me they had chickens running in and out of the house and I said they had to stop that. Well, I think the way I did it offended them, and they didn't come back for a long time.

"Later on they had a girl who was born with a terrible bilateral cleft palate. They got into a conflict with the neonatologist. One thing led to another, and they called the department of human resources because they thought the child was going home to an unsafe environment. They all called me, and I agreed to consult with them, to take responsibility more or less, if the hospital released the baby.

"I was more diplomatic in working with the family this time, but I was also clear about what the child needed. They did everything. We got the Shriners involved to repair the cleft palate. And you know, they really never even mentioned that it was a serious problem for them. They accepted this child from the start. They thought she was beautiful. The story is not over with this child. But it's clear to me that these parents accept her in ways that other parents may not. They are willing to work with me. It looks good so far.

"What I realized is that if your goal is to help your patients, then you can't ostracize them. You have to love them and accept them as they are. I tell my patients right out that I really do care what happens to them. They need to hear it.

"I'm still tough when I have to be. Sometimes the people here call me Mom. Other times I'm sure they call me something else. I know that people say, 'Watch out for that Dr. Raulerson. She's good, but if you don't do what you're supposed to do, she'll get after you.'

"This is a pretty gritty job sometimes. There's a lot of drug use in poor rural areas, and we're no exception. I was the first doctor to ever make a child abuse report in this county. It was a case in which the child was born with fetal alcohol syndrome. Three weeks before the baby was born, the mother was diagnosed with gonorrhea. The judge asked if, in my opinion, the baby would be endangered in the home. I said yes.

"I guess the main thing in this relationship we have with our patients is to be honest, be firm about what you can tolerate, and to understand as much as you can about where the patient is in their life. When we have a serious case, we focus on having a really good outcome. But you can't have a good outcome if you lose the trust of the patient or the family, and they walk away.

"A good example is this family who brought a child in because it had been bitten. The mother explained that he was playing with this rat and then it turned around and bit him. She then reaches into her diaper bag, pulls this thing out—I'm pretty sure it was a mouse—to show me. Now, I could have gotten all upset, made a big deal about it, and frightened her away for good. Instead I treated the child and we talked pretty calmly about why it's not a good idea for her son to play with rats, and why she should stop it the next time. She's continuing to rely on me, and that means I can continue to help her and her child. That's a pretty good outcome.

"Because I do care very much about my patients and I let them know it, I do open myself up for some personal pain. The hardest thing is when the outcome is not good, and there's nothing you can do. Often it happens when people seem to have everything in the world going for them. It's like God chooses the burden only for someone who can handle it. It's not the extremely poor person, but the one that should be making it through life okay. That's why I say there's no typical family, no way to predict from appearances how things are going to go.

"There was a couple in town that I liked very much. They were very good people. What they went through, and what I went through with them, was grueling.

"It started with their first daughter, who seemed to be normal but then got very sick. She didn't really develop normally. It seemed like something like Tay Sachs [a fatal disease that retards a child's growth], but that wasn't it. She was developmentally disabled, though, and the prognosis was very poor. She died when she was just a few years old.

"Later the same mother had twins which were premature. They were critically ill. One died in the hospital. The other came home. They gave her the name Hannah, and for a while she seemed beautiful. Everything went normally for a while, but then I began to see that she was going the same way. We had never found the real cause of this illness, and we never would, but the mother just tried to ignore the fact that it was happening, to have as much time with her child as she could.

"Anyway, when I finally got the chance to examine her and determine that yes, it was happening again, I just started crying. The parents were wonderful. They said, 'It's okay, Dr. Raulerson. We know, and it's okay.' Hannah lived 'til age three. We sent lab work all over the country, but we never found out what it was that she had.

"The parents tried to carry on. They adopted three children, and I thought they were going to make it. I cared so much for them. But in the end, they got divorced. I think about them once in a while. It's all part of the work, I guess. You do everything you can, and then you have to accept the outcome. It's hard though."

"Res" Girl, M.D.

෴

Bernadette Freeland-Hyde, M.D., 38, pediatrician,
Scottsdale, Arizona

Winnie Holmes, 30, teacher's aide,
Phoenix, Arizona

෴

PATIENT

Like Dr. Freeland-Hyde, Winnie Holmes grew up on the wind-swept Navajo Reservation in Northern Arizona. She met Dr. Freeland-Hyde in the weeks after her baby, Maria, was born.

She now depends on Freeland-Hyde's clinic for routine pediatric care.

"I think the biggest thing is that she is so patient with me. Maria is my only child. She has changed everything in my life. Dr. Freeland-Hyde is willing to stay there and answer everything for me.

"When she examines my daughter she doesn't do anything that different from other doctors, except for the fact that Maria doesn't seem to mind at all. I mean, Dr. Freeland-Hyde seems to have a really good way of being with babies. She's very gentle. She looks right into Maria's eyes and she's immediately very calm.

"It is true that being away from the reservation and living in the city is very hard. I think that she understands what it means, in our culture, to be away from your family. On the reservation you always have someone to go to, some place to stay. Here you have so many more responsibilities, and they are all your own. There is more opportunity. There are more jobs. But there's also a lot more pressure.

"When I go with Maria to see Dr. Freeland-Hyde I feel like I am seeing an aunt, or some other relative who is glad to see me and happy to spend the time talking about Maria.

"Her openness, and the fact that she still identifies with being a 'res' girl, makes people more comfortable. I mean, a lot of Indian people don't know how to approach someone like a doctor. First they worry about not being able to speak very well. Then there's all this worry about how you are going to be treated. If you think about history, it makes sense that someone would be afraid of a big bureaucracy. Look what has happened to us in the past. It's hard to trust.

"The other thing that Dr. Freeland-Hyde might be is a role model. She's like us, but she went to school and became a doctor, and she's very good at it. That's the kind of future I want my daughter to have. I'm glad she has a doctor who can be an example for her."

DOCTOR

Even though Bernadette Freeland was the top student at her high school on the Navajo Reservation in the Southwest, her secret dream of becoming a doctor would have seemed farfetched to those who knew she was about to become a single mother. As far as anyone knew, there was only one Navajo doctor around, and he hadn't been forced to compete for medical school and residencies while caring for a baby.

Freeland, who would later marry and become Bernadette Freeland-Hyde, could count on her family's support to see her through. With the help of a special high school teacher she applied and was accepted at Notre Dame for undergraduate studies. While her own parents raised her son, she went on to medical school at the University of Arizona and residencies in pediatrics in San Diego and Houston. Today she practices at an Indian community health clinic in Phoenix. She's the physician for a program that treats only young Indian mothers and their babies.

.   .   .

"I was born and raised around Window Rock, on the reservation. My dad was a road engineer and my mom worked in accounting. I had a sister and two brothers and a huge extended family. My mom had ten brothers and sisters.

"When I was young I think there was one Navajo doctor, Taylor Mckenzie, but we never saw him. Like everyone else, we got our medical care from the federal Indian Health Services. In the 1960s, they were mostly young doctors who were trying to get out of going in the service and being sent to Vietnam. We also thought that some of them were rejects from the white world. All of them came with the idea that it would be eighteen months and they would go.

"My earliest memory of them is that they yelled a lot at the old people, which upset me a lot. It's possible that they had to yell because the old people were deaf and they were trying to be understood. But I didn't know about that then. I just thought there was no respect there and it was terrible.

"When I was about eight years old, I had a bike accident and broke a tooth. I remember then that the main thing the dentist did was complain about being called in for an emergency. Now he was the dentist on call that day, but he still didn't like it, and he let us know it. I cried.

"Then when I was eighteen, and my son was born, the nurse was talking to the doctor about my baby's billirubin level, which was very high, and they were acting like I would never understand something so technical. Well, you know, I realized that the work they were doing was not that hard. I thought to myself 'I could do that.' And maybe I could do it better, at least when it came to being with the people. I wanted to do that, to be a doctor for people who let them know that I cared.

. . .

"There is a Navajo saying: 'A smile from a baby is like a gift from the gods.' In my culture children are really special. Traditionally they were completely indulged until about age three or four. Then you are required to take responsibility little by little. Everyone in the family is to be useful. Everyone plays an important part. It gives you a sense of who you really are.

"One thing that other doctors may not realize is that in the 1930s, '40s, and '50s we lost a lot of the connections to that tradition. A great many young children were taken away from their families and put in boarding schools. The children grew up to be parents who had lost touch with the traditional ways of raising children. They hadn't experienced it themselves. We lost a lot of the good knowledge base we once had. This is why we have a pretty high rate of abuse and neglect, and too much domestic violence. Parents don't know what to do.

"I went back to the elders and talked to them about family life. They told me a lot of it is focused on cycles, like the seasons or the day. Sunrise, for example, is the most important and powerful part of the day. You are supposed to ask the gods for help in the things you intend to do with your day. It's a good way to focus your life, to be intentional rather than just drifting. There's also a strong emphasis on respect for yourself and respect for elders.

"So many of our people live in cities now, like Phoenix, and they don't have any connection to the community. I have become not an elder exactly, but like an aunt who educates them, answers all the questions. I would say that's the biggest role I have. Indian mothers don't have the community support that they used to have. So I have to educate from the moment I walk in the door.

. . .

"Of course, they have to trust you first, and that's where I some-times use what I guess is called self-disclosure. My experience as an eighteen-year-old mother is not that different from what the mothers in my practice are going through. I let my mother raise my son while I went off to college. That was extremely painful for me. My son is now twenty and he knows about this and it's a real issue between us. He's gone through some pretty hard times and I feel bad about it. But it all means that I know something about what these young mothers are going through. When I let them know about myself, I can see them start to trust me. I am a 'res' girl just like them.

"Most of the parenting issues are the same that anyone deals with. Sleep is a big one. I explain to them how to help a child learn how to settle herself down and sleep. Rocking a baby to sleep is not a good idea because they won't learn to comfort themselves. Everyone needs to know about feeding and toilet training. Later on bed-wetting can be a big one. I try to reassure parents and children. Most of the time what they are going through is normal. Most moms do a very good job.

"But it doesn't always work out. Families can be confusing to me, and I'm not always really patient. I had a four- or five-year-old come in with severe asthma. She was with the stepmom. Well, she didn't know anything about the medication the child was supposed to take. She didn't know how often, how much, even what kind it was.

"Well, I try to be diplomatic, but I wasn't this time. I said, 'You know, asthma can be fatal if you don't take care of it.' This is true, and we do see a lot of asthma. And it can be managed best when the patient and the parents know everything in detail about how the disease works and how the medicines work.

"But I could have been much gentler, and this lady let me know it. She wrote me a letter that said she had just met this child and that she hadn't been told anything about the asthma. Believe me, I haven't done anything like that since. I don't mention death like that in relation to asthma anymore, either.

"As you practice medicine you learn from your mistakes, and you learn what your strengths are, too. As time goes by, I find myself making strong connections to my home. I acknowledge that I sometimes still feel insecure in the white man's world. I know a lot of the mothers I see feel that way, too. But I also know who I am, and I respect my identity. And I will use anything from my culture that I think will work, including Indian ceremonies.

"I had one family who came to me because their twelve-year-old boy was having a lot of adolescent problems. He was extremely disobedient, and it really looked like he could get himself into some serious trouble. He tried counseling, but that failed, and I really concluded that Western medicine was not helping him. I told them that I thought an Indian ceremony would help. The ceremony has a very powerful effect on people. You say things out loud, in front of others, and it changes things. It touches people very profoundly. They used it, and it worked. I have since tried it with myself and my own son, the one I didn't raise, and I think it has helped us, too.

"When Indian people find out that I respect Indian culture

as much as Western medicine, they invest even more trust in me. One of my favorite patients was a ten-year-old boy I saw when I worked in a clinic in San Diego. He was being raised just by his father, who was fifty or older. His father really paid attention to his son's asthma.

"This child was on a great many medicines. He also had attention deficit disorder, which meant he could respond in some unexpected way to changes in his medicine. But they trusted me to keep experimenting with doses and different kinds of medicines. By the time we were done, he was down to one or two.

"I think that success happened because I am open and I am supportive of people in the community. I am willing to show who I am. I am both a 'res' girl and a doctor, and that puts people at ease. I think that's why I get along so well with these mothers and their babies."

PART FOUR

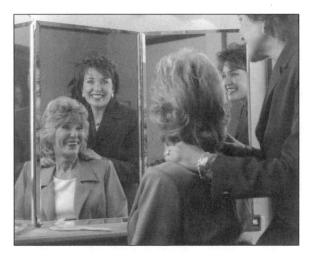

Dr. Lori Hansen

The

Healers

More Than Skin Deep

↝

*Lori Hansen, M.D., 44, facial plastic surgeon,
Oklahoma City, Oklahoma*

*Helen Luketich, 46, homemaker,
Leander, Texas*

↝

PATIENT

The lowest moment in Helen Luketich's first marriage came in the split second that her husband kicked her in the stomach. Her injuries were so severe that she went to the hospital where an emergency hysterectomy was performed. She was twenty-one years old.

Through fifteen years in the same marriage, Luketich suffered broken bones, internal injuries, and innumerable cuts and bruises on her face. Ashamed and afraid, she was unable to leave the relationship until a friend, who was also a battered wife, literally coached her into freedom.

Though she had left the violence behind, Luketich was reminded of it every time she looked in the mirror. The physical beatings, emotional torture, and years of depression had turned her face into a lined, careworn image. She could have passed for sixty-five, or even seventy years old. Some employers rejected her job applications because they thought she wasn't vigorous. Others believed she couldn't serve the public. She became convinced that her future held only struggle in low-paying jobs and social isolation.

"I became Dr. Hansen's patient in a pretty unusual way. I had been asked to be on a TV show about battered women. One part of the show was about a program that some plastic surgeons had started to help women like me. Dr. Lori was on the show and she offered me her services, for free, right there on television. Of course I said yes. There wasn't any question in my mind.

"The thing about Dr. Lori is that even though she's very beautiful on the outside, what you really notice the most is how beautiful she is on the inside. Her whole being radiates a sense of caring. That came through the first time I went to her office. We talked about my life and how it showed on my face. I had scars over both my eyes and over my lip. I told her I had once been asked if I was the mother of a fifty-two-year-old woman I was with. We both cried.

"I think Dr. Lori really understands how women feel about how they look. We all want to be pretty. We can't help it. But it's more than skin deep, and she knows that, too. When you don't feel like you look good, it really affects your self-esteem. I remember she told me that she was the same age that I was and that it wasn't right that I had to live the way I was living. It wasn't about my looks as much as it was about how I felt. One thing that she noticed, and I had to agree with her, was that I never really smiled. I don't think I had smiled for a long, long time.

"It's hard to describe how good they make you feel in Dr. Lori's office. When I went for the surgery it was cold. They met me with heated blankets and an old-fashioned comforter. They took the fear right out of me. Then Dr. Lori came in and said, 'Are you ready to be beautiful?'

"As we were getting ready, I remember that I kept pulling my hair over my ears. Dr. Lori stopped and asked me if there was anything that we hadn't talked about that I would like her to do something about. Well, my ex-husband had pulled on my ears a lot and they were very large. I asked her if she could fix them and she said that was no problem. She did it right then.

"Of course it didn't stop with the surgery. That night I went back to my hotel room and a nurse came over from the office to bring me medication. On the second night Dr. Lori stopped in herself. She knew I would be feeling a little low, and she gave me a big hug and said everything would be alright.

"When they finally took all the bandages off, what I saw was just amazing. Dr. Lori had given me my smile back. She had also given me back my independence. I was able to go get a much better job in real estate, where I work with the public every day. I have a lot more confidence. I have a wonderful second husband and grandchildren. I have the motivation to try for things in life and really enjoy being with people. Dr. Lori gave me these things. I will always be grateful to her for it."

DOCTOR

Dr. Hansen was born in Colorado and grew up on a wheat farm outside the small town of Southaven, Kansas. After medical school she did a residency in plastic surgery in Birmingham, Alabama, and undertook additional training in head and neck plastic surgery at a private clinic in Beverly Hills, California. In a field dominated by men, Dr. Hansen is not just a rare female, but also the only country's facial plastic surgeon to be a veteran of the Miss America pageant. While in medical school, she was selected to be Miss Oklahoma.

"Most of my work, I'd say 90–95 percent, is making people look better. The rest is repairing scars and other injuries, or helping someone after cancer. I recently built a new nose for an older woman whose nose had been destroyed by cancer. When the Oklahoma City bombing occurred I was also involved in the repair of some wounds, but there was not a lot of that actually, because either people were slightly injured or they were killed."

Dr. Hansen will admit she prefers work that enables her to help people look better rather than reconstructive surgery. "There's a certain art to it that I really enjoy. I am meticulous, kind of a perfectionist, and I like improving imperfections. People do suffer, they are treated differently, if they are not attractive or they feel they are not. It's a fact of life in our society. Like it or not, people, especially women, are affected very seriously by how they look. When they come to me saying they are having a problem, I take it seriously.

"If you want proof that appearance is very important to how people feel about themselves, then you just have to look at some of the women we have treated in our program for people who have been victims of abuse. One of these patients was held down by her husband who then burned her face with cigarettes. Others have been abused for so long that they show it in their faces. They look beaten down. Some are offered senior citizens' discounts when they are only forty-five. They have trouble getting accepted by others, even getting a job.

"After surgery these women are younger and brighter looking and they feel more confident, too. Helen Luketich is a wonderful example. She had eyelid surgery and a face-lift. She's now a very successful businesswoman in real estate. If you want an example of how what they call cosmetic surgery helps people, that's one.

"Another good example is the military officer who was having trouble getting any further promotions because he thought he looked too old. Not long after he had some work done he was promoted.

"I think the most important thing for me to do in my relationship with patients is to understand what their expectations really are, and help them be realistic both about what kind of work they can do and what the result will be. These women—most still are women—don't need someone telling them they are wrong about this and that. They need someone to look in the mirror with them, study their face, and listen.

"On the first visit we sit and look in the mirror, and I ask them to give me their priorities. When I first started I made the mistake of letting a patient ask me first what I thought they needed, and then answering them. I said something about their face that they hadn't ever been aware of. Maybe it was about getting a chin implant when what they really came in for was to have work done on their nose. I made things much worse, not better.

"So now I will only start with a patient's wishes. Usually they are able to point directly to the thing they want done, and I am able to see what it is and we proceed from there. But sometimes you get a patient who really can't point to anything serious. You'll adjust the mirror this way and that, put all different lighting on their face, and you can't see it. I had one young woman who was upset because one nostril was slightly larger than the other. Obviously she didn't need plastic surgery.

"In other cases I may see what a patient is talking about, but because I'm a woman, because I know where they are coming from and I know a lot about how to make yourself look good from my pageant days, I can give them advice that saves them from going through surgery.

"I recently had an older patient who fit into this category. She wanted something to make her face look younger. But all she really needed to look attractive as a woman her age was appropriate makeup and maybe a hair extension. She very much wanted surgery but we wouldn't do it, and I think that was the right decision.

"I also try to assess my patients to make sure they are not so narcissistic that they are truly disturbed. Those are patients that you really cannot help. They will never be satisfied, so you are much better off not treating them and putting your time and energy into someone you can actually help.

"Once you and a patient have come to an agreement to do some surgery you have to establish a shared idea of what will happen. I have to be able to acknowledge what their concerns are and affirm them, otherwise I have no credibility, and we don't share the same starting point.

"Then we establish realistic expectations. One of my colleagues was sued by a patient who had rhinoplasty because she was sure he had made her nose crooked. Well, the truth was that he did a pretty good surgery, and it was unrealistic for the patient to expect much better. The patient wasn't clear on what the outcome would be, and that's where the problem happened.

"Cases like that are another example of why I try to get to know my patients very well. I'm not just fixing their face. I am sharing their life. I ask them about their ideas of what is beautiful and what their feelings about their appearance may be. The truth is that I don't think of myself as beautiful. I think that if I put my makeup on and dress well I can look good.

"But I have the same insecurities that all women have, even though I competed for Miss America. And if you don't think I'm affected by how society demands that women look beautiful, you're wrong. I have patients remind me of this many times when they see me before or after surgery. I'm in my scrubs. I don't have any makeup on. And the patient will say to her family, 'You know, normally she looks much better than this.'

"I remind women that an absolutely perfect face is not interesting and won't be noticed. One Miss Universe I know of had such a perfect face that she wound up modeling for Sears because they don't want the models to be noticed. I'm not sure that's the kind of beauty most women are looking for, not being noticed.

"In the end, when I've really done my job well, a patient who has appropriate surgery will actually be able to forget about her face—stop worrying about appearance—and focus instead on living a life. That's the real purpose of the surgery, and I think my patients know that I understand their feelings and want to get them to that point where they feel good about themselves and can move on."

Faith, Hope, and Medicine

❦

Ivonne Jimenez, M.D., 29, internist,
Bayamon, Puerto Rico

Angeles Caceres, 73, retired teacher,
Carolina, Puerto Rico

❦

PATIENT

Angeles Caceres was one of eight children born and raised in
Carolina. Her father owned a little grocery store. Her mother
was a homemaker. Now retired, she lives with her husband Jose,

a former chef, in a whitewashed bungalow in a quiet section of the city where she was born.

Mrs. Caceres' first physician was a general practitioner who was, literally, the only doctor in the neighborhood. She recalls him as competent, but aloof. She had always hoped to find a doctor who would be both a healer and a friend. She says she found this in Dr. Ivonne Jimenez, an internist she first met in 1996.

"My family doctor was on vacation when I noticed a little lump in my breast. I made an appointment with a doctor I had heard about and went to the building where his office was. But I wasn't sure. I was looking around and I saw Dr. Jimenez' office and stopped in. It was just a feeling I had, that this woman doctor might be the one for me. The nurse said she would see me that day, but I wasn't really prepared for that. I like to take a shower, be very prepared before I go to any doctor. I made an appointment for the next week.

"I was a little afraid when I went back, but when she came out I knew she was the right one. She was very open, very warm. She called me Doña Angeles, which is a sign of respect, and listened very carefully to me. On the forms she gave me I wrote 'retired teacher' under occupation. She said her mother was a retired teacher too.

"That first time she spent a lot of time with me. The only focus, the only thing in the world that she cared about was me. I felt that way every time afterward. She would study my laboratory test results one-by-one with me, going over each one. Other doctors just look at it quickly and say 'You're fine.'

Dr. Jimenez was much more careful. She paid very close attention to how I was doing.

"She was very respectful during the examination, but when she felt the lump she said that it would be a good idea to do a biopsy. She said she was concerned, but she also acted like it was not such a big, difficult problem that we couldn't handle it. She found me a surgeon she thought would be very good for me, and he was.

"I was afraid going to that first appointment, but with Dr. Jimenez I wasn't afraid after that. I have a lot of faith, and she does too. It comes though when you're with her. She believes that everything is going to work out for the best, that God has a plan, and that makes you feel calmer.

"When the results came back we had to make a choice; lumpectomy with chemo, or a radical mastectomy and possibly no chemo. I had seen a friend go through chemotherapy and it was awful. But I am also vain, like anyone. Puerto Ricans may be the most vain people in the world. But this is my health we're talking about—cancer. So I chose the radical. My vanity is not so great that I would choose something else.

"Before the surgery she came to see me in the hospital. She wasn't doing the operation. She didn't have any other patients in that hospital. But she came because she was thinking of me, and she gave me a book of prayers. I had the peace of God when I finally went into the operating room. I felt extremely peaceful.

"Dr. Jimenez never stopped caring about me. She came to see me on the day after the operation, and she called me on the phone every day after that until our next appointment. Every time she talks to me first like a friend. She asks about my family. Then we talk about my health. After the operation I didn't have to go through chemo, which was a blessing. They gave me that new drug, Tamoxifen, and I have been fine ever since.

"Dr. Jimenez referred me to a surgeon and an oncologist who were both a lot like her. They were very warm, very caring. They all understood that I have very strong religious faith and they were respectful. They all opened their hearts to me. That's what makes them special. And to think I found them all because I walked in a different door on the day I was going to the doctor. I think the Lord was involved in that decision."

DOCTOR

Like Angeles Caceres, Dr. Ivonne Jimenez was the daughter of a neighborhood shopkeeper. As a preschooler she accompanied her schoolteacher mother to her classroom, where she was enrolled in first grade at age four. Her first physician role model was a cousin who was a practicing surgeon. Jimenez was trained at the University of Puerto Rico School of Medicine, where she is now an instructor. Her residencies included the study of gerontology at Mount Sinai Hospital in New York City.

"My cousin was the kind of doctor who saw a lot of patients for free. He did a lot of trauma work. People would come into the hospital, and he would do whatever was needed without thinking about getting paid. I remember him saying that the one thing he hoped that all his patients would do is say, 'Thank you.' It actually hurt him when they didn't.

"I saw him as a patient just one time. I was fifteen, and I had discovered a lump in my breast. When you are fifteen this is very embarrassing, the idea of being examined by anyone. But he was wonderful. He asked my mother to come in, and he had a nurse there too. He draped every part of my body except where he had to examine me, and he talked to me the whole time. He was always a very charming person, easy to talk to. But he knew his stuff, medically. It gave you a lot of confidence.

"In my case, the lump turned out to be nothing. In those days they often removed them anyway, and he did. The thing that I remembered from that experience is the helplessness and the fear. I felt very scared going in for surgery. The place was very cold and I felt very alone. No matter what kind of procedure you go in for, surgery is frightening.

"In our training at medical school we learned to have empathy for our patients. I go in and I ask a patient one open-ended question. 'How can I help you today?' Then I listen as carefully as I can. I am not distant or emotionally cold. There is a risk with this way of doing things. If something bad happens to your patient, if one dies, then I suffer. But this is what being a doctor is.

"When Doña Angeles came in for the first time I could tell that she was afraid. I wanted to be like a friend and a professional who could help her feel less afraid. One of the most important things I can do for someone in that situation is make sure they know we have a lot of treatment options, and they are not in a hopeless situation. I then put a lot of thought into finding a surgeon who was right for her—very kind, gentle—and I made the phone call to his office. I did that because I was worried that Angeles would not be assertive enough and they would give her an appointment a month away. A lot of patients have doctors in the family or know a surgeon to call. She did not, but she still needed to be seen immediately.

"Most patients are not so emergent. I see mostly older people, and many of them come in with multiple problems that they have not been able to fix with other doctors. Usually it's quite clear they are depressed. I ask if they have been crying, if they are lonely, if they are eating or sleeping well. If they answer these questions in a way that makes it seem they are depressed, I ask them to take a written assessment test.

"The test helps a lot of people who might not otherwise be open to the idea that they are depressed to see what's going on. But in some cases I run into what is a religious belief that it's wrong to feel depressed, that they are somehow defying God if they are not happy with the life He gave them.

"I have a pretty strong religious faith myself and it's times like these when I'll let a patient know that. I point out to them that there are many examples of depressed people in the Bible. They are surprised to hear that, but I can tell them about people like the prophet Elias. When it didn't rain for years the people asked him to pray for rain and it worked. God answered his prayer, but in the Bible it says he sat under a tree and cried. God then made him sleep and sent angels to bring him food. Then he got better.

"If I share this story with some patients, and let them know that I understand their religious feelings and I have faith too, they often become more receptive. This isn't something I always do. In fact, in general I'm pretty private about my life. But when people are open with me about their beliefs I feel it's okay for me to be open with them. It helps us feel closer to each other.

.   .   .

"Religious faith is an important cultural consideration with a lot of patients. I am comfortable with that. I believe that miraculous things happen. I have seen them. I had one patient who had a kidney tumor and was scheduled for surgery. The tumor was there. She prayed for three weeks and when she went back, it was gone. I've seen the pictures. It's there and then it's not.

"This is why I don't believe in telling patients how much time they have left. They can be told they are seriously sick and what is happening to them. But miracles do happen, and I'm not going to take that possibility away from anyone. I've seen cases of older people in renal failure that we wouldn't think could make it through the night, and then they go home. A few weeks ago a patient of mine had a brain hemorrhage and was almost comatose. We were considering neurosurgery when all of a sudden he recovers completely.

"This is what makes me think that faith and hope are part of healing. I am like a coach with patients, telling them they can do it, helping their bodies recover, and supporting them."

Good Karma

⤸

Ajay Berdia, M.D., 38, neurologist,
Long Island, New York

Elizabeth Allyn, 17, student,
Long Island, New York

⤸

PATIENT

In their acute stages meningitis and encephalitis can be life-threatening and even mild cases may drag on for months. They can also leave a patient with mysterious, long-term neurologi-

cal illnesses that are difficult to diagnose and treat. Elizabeth
Allyn met Ajay Berdia, M.D., when, months after she was supposedly cured of her illnesses, she developed a kind of sleeping
sickness.

"Two years ago I was diagnosed with meningitis and encephalitis. It was probably caused by a virus. It was in the summer. I got
sick at a music camp I was going to. The main thing was that I
slept a lot, more than twenty hours a day sometimes. I was very
disoriented and I had a lot of trouble sleeping. I was very sick for
a summer, but then got better.

"After I thought I was all better I started having these new
episodes. It felt sort of like the encephalitis was coming back. I
would get very tired and sleep all day. When I was awake, I really
wasn't myself. I couldn't focus on conversations, read, or even
watch TV. I was disoriented, afraid, even pretty paranoid. This
was totally new to me. It was horrible. I missed a lot of school.
And I was scared I was losing my mind.

"We had a really hard time figuring out what was going on
with me. None of my regular doctors could say what it was, and
I was finally referred to a psychiatrist. She didn't think it was
really a psychiatric problem. She said that she thought I should
see a neurologist, that was Dr. Berdia.

"In the beginning, Dr. Berdia struck me as someone who
was very gentle. He listened very carefully to everything I said.
This helped, because I was feeling like I was a really strange person, that no one would understand how hard this all was for me.
I kept missing a lot of school, and my thinking was very fuzzy. It
was really bad.

"At first Dr. Berdia didn't have any idea what was wrong with me, but he agreed that it was a real problem, that it was serious, and that someone should try to figure it out.

"He thought it might be some kind of strange seizure disorder. He gave me anti-seizure medication. But since he didn't know for sure that's what it was, he sent me for a PET scan. This was something he had to really fight for me to get, because it's a very expensive test. It showed my brain was normal, but in the frontal lobes there was some decreased activity.

"Unfortunately, this didn't give us an answer and the episodes kept happening. Every few months I'd get sick for a week. He wanted to see me when it was happening. But it was hard because there was nothing anyone could do. At the hospital he would hold my hand; he asked if I wanted anything to eat and ran to get me some cookies. I was too out of it to really appreciate all that he was doing to show that he cared. But again the tests really didn't show anything.

"He had a lot of faith in my parents. They did a lot of research and kept on top of things. So did he. Finally when my mom suggested it might be Kleine-Levin syndrome, which she had heard about, he agreed. He was happy that an answer was found, but a little upset that he didn't find it. But this is a very rare thing. It only affects about one hundred people in the country. We got some medication.

"The truth is, he hasn't cured me, but he has been able to listen to me in a way that other medical professionals haven't. It makes me feel better having someone agree that this is a real problem.

"Because I had this experience, I'm hoping to go into neurology when I grow up. He's a warm, caring doctor. He really genuinely cares about what happens to you and how you feel. He advocated for me. He pushed for me. He made me feel like I mattered. I was validated. And he tried.

"He cared about me as a person, not just a patient. He wanted to know who I was besides just a girl with a strange neurological disorder. He talked to me about nose rings and my flowered boots. He is a scientist with humanity.

"Once, when they were giving me a hard time at school about absences, I was told to get a doctor's note. I went right to his office. He made time for me in the middle of his day. And when I told him I was worried he might not give me the note he said, 'I don't work for the gym teachers. I work for you.' That made me feel like he was really my doctor. He was there for me."

DOCTOR

Dr. Ajay Berdia's faith plays a strong role in his commitment to patients. He says that a life of service is a positive expression of Hindu beliefs, and that in his relationships with patients he hopes to create *duah* or spiritual good will.

Born and raised in Bombay by his grandparents, Dr. Berdia's father is a surgeon who practiced first in England and then in North Carolina. Ajay Berdia joined his parents in the United States after high school. He says that the long separation from his parents helped him to appreciate the importance of close relationships.

.   .   .

"I can tell you when I really started to understand about the doctor-patient relationship and what I can do to make it positive. It happened during my residency in neurology at Syracuse University Hospital. It was probably in my first two weeks. A guy came into the emergency room in a wheelchair. The attending, Dr. Jack Wolfe, told me, 'He's an MS [multiple sclerosis] patient and he's come here to die. He's your patient.'

"Now when I went to see this patient he was very aware of where he was. He was eating. He was breathing well. He had no heart condition. I thought he was fine, and I couldn't understand what they meant by saying he was there to die. I told this all to Dr. Wolfe and said I was going to give him some steroids and get him going. He said, 'Okay, Ajay, he's your patient.'

"Everything went fine until one day they called me because he was unresponsive. We were able to bring him back, but from that day on he went downhill. I remember going to Dr. Wolfe and saying, 'I'm coming to you for direction.' He would say, 'Ajay, take care of him.' I could not figure out what he meant by that.

"Well, when he became unresponsive a second time we worked very hard to revive him again. I shocked him. But he died because he just couldn't breathe any more. That's what the MS finally did to him. It stopped his breathing.

"Three days later I go into Dr. Wolfe's office and he has this patient's brain in a jar on his desk. He asks me, 'Ajay, what have you learned?' I couldn't answer. I was completely confused. Then he showed me the plaques that had developed in the brain right in the area that controlled his breathing. It was obvious, as I held my patient's brain in my hand, that the disease had taken him, and it had been inevitable.

"What I learned was that I hadn't recognized what was really happening to the person I was treating. He was dying. It was undeniable. But I hadn't faced that. I had tried to stop the cycle of nature. I had never even talked with him about the fact that he was dying. He knew it, but I didn't respect that. In the end I had made all kinds of efforts and even mutilated his body so he could live a few more days and die anyway. I had treated death as an enemy, instead of part of life. I felt sorry for the patient and sorry for me. I had missed an opportunity to really connect with him and help him as a person.

"I have never forgotten this experience. It affects how I deal with patients like that. It's important because neurologists get a lot of calls to determine if a patient is really brain dead, or if they have a chance for recovery. It's the neurologist who has to make the determination.

"Today, for example, I had to tell a family that the father was so brain damaged that he was not going to recover. They had to make a decision on withdrawing life support and I had to tell them the truth. I went in. I talked very respectfully to the patient, using his name even though he was not able to respond. I treated the body with a great deal of respect.

"But when I was finished I told them the truth, which was that the person they knew was already gone. This was something they were able to understand. They cried, and I cried too. I can't help that, and I don't try to stop it. It's natural. But then they had to make the decision, and they did let him go, let him die.

.   .   .

"With Elizabeth I started out trying to make her comfortable. She came in with her parents, and I wanted her to know that she was in charge. I was her doctor, and I was going to pay close attention to what she felt and what she had to say. I made her the big person in the room. I put her in charge. Sometimes when a person is resistant to taking an active role I will ask them to sit in my chair, behind the desk. That puts them in the position of authority. And they are the authority. They are the patient.

"In cases where you have trouble making a diagnosis I make sure the patient knows that I truly care about what is happening, that I believe they have something real, and that I will do everything I can. I will take whatever information is available, and I will collaborate. In this case the parents came up with some information that was very important. They were better doctors than me. But what I was able to do was remain open-minded so that I could help them better. If I had ignored what they were discovering I would not have been a very good doctor at all. I am not here to be right. I am not here to be the god of medicine. I am here to help.

"The idea of *duah* is that good will, service to others, builds good will toward you. A patient who thinks good things about me, it's like having money in the bank, spiritually. I believe the soul is on a journey to high levels, and that positive energy— those good vibes—are all part of it. The way you act here con- tributes to what people say is your karma.

"Good relationships with patients, showing respect, being

honest, is also something that just makes your life as a doctor so much better. The idea of medicine is not to figure out ways to get what's in someone else's pocket into yours. Help people. That's all that's required. Just help them any way you can."

Never Met a Patient
He Didn't Like

↬

Calvin Martin, M.D., 71, general practice,
Arcadia, Florida

George Bellamy, 65, retired banker,
Arcadia, Florida

↬

PATIENT

Born in the era before antibiotics, George Bellamy's earliest memories of doctors revolve around two country physicians who made housecalls in the hill country of East Tennessee. They had little to offer in terms of medications, but their presence was considered healing. "They had a stethoscope and a thermometer, but mostly they just told you what to expect when you were sick and that everything would be all right."

George Bellamy has been a patient of Dr. Calvin Martin since 1964. Dr. Martin has been the Bellamy family's physician, delivering two children and diagnosing everything from allergies to heart disease.

"The thing about Dr. Martin is that when you are with him, you feel like you are the center of the universe. I mean, I don't think he's met a person that he doesn't like. But when you are with him the focus is all on you. He doesn't forget what you told him the last time and he always follows up on it. You feel like this very intelligent man really cares about you, and he's going to use everything he's got to help you. That's a very good feeling.

"This concern is not just something he puts on. He really is your friend. I remember once he made a house call because I was having some chest pain. He said he thought I should go to the hospital, and he put me in the car and drove me over himself. It turned out that it wasn't a heart attack. It was myocarditis. But he wanted to be sure and I really appreciated that.

"But the most important thing is that he knows his stuff. In 1989 we did a stress test. He made me stop right in the middle of it. He diagnosed me with heart trouble right on the spot and sent me straight to a hospital in Sarasota. I had an angioplasty the next day.

"I don't mean to say that Dr. Martin thinks he knows it all. That's not a good idea for anybody, and he'll refer you to a specialist as soon as he reaches the limit of what he can do. But if he can help you, he will. When it was decided my daughter needed allergy shots, he was able to give them. I remember once I dropped her off for the shots and forgot to go back and get her. When I finally did, they had her working in the back office putting files away. She loved it, and she always was happy to go to the doctor after that.

"I guess the point is, Dr. Martin makes you feel comfortable. He becomes part of your life, and it's natural and relaxed. I've told him many times that even though he's older than me, he's got to stick around to sign my death certificate when the time comes. I don't want anybody else to take care of me in the end."

DOCTOR

Dr. Calvin Martin's father and father-in-law were both small-town doctors in prewar Florida. In them he saw examples of both effective and failing doctor-patient relationships. His father, brilliant, gruff, and often impatient, provided examples of what he would not do. His father-in-law, who took pleasure in his patients and respected even their folk remedies, was a model of positive interactions.

After medical school at the University of Tennessee and residency in Columbus, Georgia, Dr. Martin began practice in Arcadia in 1960. Then, the town was still a quiet agricultural center beside the Peace River. Today it is a mecca for retirees. His patients include many who have seen him for more than thirty years and others who only recently moved to one of the many local retirement communities. In his relationships with patients he emphasizes offering them full attention, respecting their own feelings about their conditions, and understanding their customs and culture.

"The first time I really saw clearly how powerful your relationship with the patient can be—and how important honesty is—was during my residency. We had this one patient, a man, who had cancer of the lung. He threw things at the residents and yelled at the nurses. He was horrible.

"The thing was, his wife would not tell him that he had cancer, and she didn't want us to tell him either. But he knew something was seriously wrong. He knew he was dying, but everyone else was denying it.

"One day I went into his room and he just came out with it. He said, 'Have I got cancer?'

"I had to tell him the truth. He had asked me straight out. So I did. The minute he heard it he became a different man. He thanked me for telling him the truth, because he knew there was something very serious happening and resented being lied to. He was wonderful after that. He died five days later, but the end was much better because I had been truthful with him.

"That man in the hospital also taught me that the fears and anxieties we feel are based on real things. Even if a doctor cannot find the cause, the patient knows when there's something wrong. Chronic fatigue is like this. A lot of people say it's not real, but the patients know different. And sometimes you get lucky and can help. I had one woman who we put on an antiviral medication for the flu. Her chronic fatigue got much better. Now she's just on it all the time. It's treating something, so you can't say what she had was all in her imagination.

"This is the opposite of what you are taught in medical school. In medical school they tell you that 75 percent of the people you are going to see have nothing really wrong with them. That's not true. I think they all have something real, but we are just not finding it.

"Now a lot of people will say that these patients, especially the ones who seem to be always shopping for doctors, are hypochondriacs. It's possible that some of what they are dealing with is psychological in nature. But there's almost always a physical part, too.

"I have a patient, Miss Farley, who fits the picture of what everyone says is a hypochondriac. Every time I see her she has a long list of complaints. She's so persistent in her complaints that she pesters everyone to death. But the fact is, she does have a form of lupus, and osteoporosis, and one doctor even took out one of her kidneys when he probably didn't have to.

"I never rejected her, but I would often have to stand there listening for thirty-five or forty minutes just to sort out her complaints. Then one day I came in very tired and I sat down next to her on the table. I was only there for three or four minutes, but she got right to the point about what was bothering her the most that day, and I was able to help her. I was so surprised by how easily it went I asked her what was different this time.

"'You actually sat down and talked to me,' she said. 'That was the difference.'

"I realized that whenever I talk with patients standing up,

they have the feeling that I'm always about to walk out on them. Sitting down for three minutes can feel like more of a connection than when I stand there for thirty.

"I also stay with them long enough to let them bring up another problem, if they have to. Consultants who advise us on working more efficiently say we should put off a patient's secondary complaints, if they aren't serious, until the next visit. But a lot of times a patient won't mention something very important, or even embarrassing, until after they've gotten comfortable with you talking about something else.

"Another thing I do is make my notes after the encounter. I do it immediately after I leave the room, so I don't forget anything or fall behind. But I never make notes as a patient is talking. That's distracting for them, and it means I'm not really giving them my full attention.

"It helps to know the culture of the patients you are treating, too. My father-in-law compiled this whole book of folk remedies that are used around here. He called them 'Cracker Cures.' They were things that had been discovered to work over the years. People would find out about them from old medicine ladies. One I recall was putting warm urine in the ear for an earache. Well, the warmth was soothing, and you know, one of the most used ear drops today has urea as an ingredient. Foxglove is digitalis.

"Knowing these things can help you avoid serious problems, too. Once I was treating a little black baby. He was very fat and came in unable to breathe. I was about to do a tracheotomy when I looked in the folds of skin on his neck and found a thread—with a dime attached to it—that had been cutting off the airway. I snipped it off and he started to breath fine.

"The snowbirds are another big part of our culture here, and I try hard to understand their situation. These are mostly older people who retire and then leave everything they know, all their friends and family, to live in paradise in a trailer in Florida. Often the problems they have are definitely affected by their isolation. They become depressed; they feel sicker. Sometimes you have to reach out to their relatives and get them to change their living situation.

"I think the advice I would give other doctors who want to have a good relationship with their patients is that they let themselves enjoy the time they spend with people. I have one patient who shares a love of guava jelly with me. Sometimes I'll come in to my office and find a jar of jelly on my desk, or maybe the most beautiful ripe pear. Another lady brings me strawberry preserves. And one of the men I see, who comes down from Buffalo every winter, brings me a kind of wine—Bully Hill—that I can't get here. I call him my rum runner. These people are my friends. I like them and I hope that they like me."

Lessons in Love

୬

Elisa Nicholas, M.D., 47,
pediatrician and director of The Children's Clinic
at Long Beach Memorial Medical Center, Long Beach, California

Norma Almarez, 43, and her four children,
Abigail, 16, Abraham, 15, Joshua, 10, and Adriana, 13,
Wilvomir, California

୬

PATIENT

Norma Almarez, 43, is the mother of four children ages 16, 15, 13, and 10. Two, 16-year-old Abigail and 15-year-old Abraham, are mentally retarded. One, 10-year-old Joshua, suffers from autism. Adriana, age 13, does not have any serious health problems. Ms. Almarez drives forty-five miles, from Temecula to Long Beach, so that her children can see Dr. Nicholas.

"We have been seeing Dr. Nicholas since 1990. Before then, we tried everything to find a doctor who was comfortable with retarded children. With retarded children you have to be very patient, but very focused on what you need to get done. Most doctors don't want to do it, or they can't. They don't have the right heart. That is why Dr. Nicholas is a blessing. She is gentle, always patient. And she cares about me, too.

"If you have three disabled children, you work very hard. I plan a day ahead, so I know what I'm going to do. And I rely on God. But the truth is, I don't always have that much faith in God. When I feel that way, I try to remind myself that God only gives me what I can manage. God believes in me, so I believe in Him.

"Dr. Nicholas understands all of this. Sometimes she will tell me that I have to take a day off for myself. It's the doctor's orders for me. But she knows I won't take a whole day, so she says, 'Go for a few hours, an afternoon.' I do, and it makes me feel so much better. I think I can come home and do better with my children, too.

"I understand that my family is different. We are not like everyone else. One of the other things that's not the same is we don't have a lot of money. But that doesn't matter to Dr. Nicholas. She treats us equal, like all the others. I am very sure that we get the same care, just as good, as any rich family. That's not true at every clinic or doctor's office, but it's true with Dr. Nicholas.

"Maybe it's because she has a son who is not perfect, too. I do know that she thinks that every child is valuable, precious. And even though she has suggested we find a doctor who is Latino, or who is closer to us, we are going to keep seeing Dr. Nicholas as long as we can. She is a very kind person, a human being. She a doctor, a mom, a worker, a friend. We're part of her and she's part of us. I pray to thank God for her."

DOCTOR

The daughter of the first child of Greek immigrants to become a doctor in Los Angeles, Elisa Nicholas has always been interested in the city's diverse cultures and communities. After training at Yale and UCLA, she practiced at hospitals and clinics around the city, serving mainly the children of poor immigrants. She went to Africa in 1985 and '86 to work in local health programs and finally settled in at Long Beach in 1988. Ten years later she is the director of a non-profit clinic that serves mainly the working poor, including large numbers of recent immigrants from Latin America, Cambodia, and other Asian countries.

Despite her training and professional experience, Dr. Nicholas finds the key to her relationships with patients in her personal life. A son born with cerebral palsy has taught her about the struggles of parents with sick children and the challenge of building a balanced life.

.   .   .

"We have a number of patients who have multiple disabilities. I let many of the parents know that I have a son with CP, Tommy, because it tells them that I understand something about what they are going through.

"I see a lot of giving. I've seen parents accept their children completely for who they are. These parents believe that God gave them their children because he knew they could handle it. He knew they would take care of these special kids. And they do. They have been examples for me, and they have helped me be a better mother and a better doctor.

"I can give you an example of how these parents feel about their children. It involves the mother of a multiply handicapped child who eventually died. This mom was the sole caretaker of this child. She arranged all the appointments, got the ambulance to bring her here, and handled everything.

"After the child died she got an appointment card in the mail. Obviously it was a mistake. But she came in to the office anyway, just to tell us how upset she was about the insensitivity of it.

"I sat with her and she said, 'I bet everyone here is saying that it was a blessing that my daughter died.'

"I told her that I thought that she must be suffering because her daughter was her whole life. She said that was true. I know that it's true, because no matter how devastated a child may be by a disability, you can always find something beautiful. They have beautiful hair, eyes, lashes, something. Her child was in a vegetative state, but that didn't matter.

"The ability these parents have to love is really impressive. I saw a mother today who already has two autistic kids and now has a new baby that she is afraid cannot see. I don't know for sure that the baby is blind, but she may be right. Now someone might say that a mother like that would be overwhelmed, but she's not. In fact, her paying job is taking care of a girl with cerebral palsy whose family ignores her. She talks to me a lot about how to help this child.

"These parents are much stronger and much wiser because they have gone through their suffering. They know what's important. I do too. I mean, I know a lot of people in my social circle who obsess about getting everything for their child and complain about not getting into the gifted class at school. Well, I have a son who had a lot of trouble just learning to walk, and I have patients who will never be able to talk to their parents.

"Hope is really important, even when as the doctor you see that there's not much reason to hope that the immediate medical situation will get any better. One example is a child I'm treating who is likely to wind up on a ventilator. She's really non-functional and it's remarkable she's lived this long.

"I haven't raised the issue of a DNR [Do Not Resusitate] order because the mother needs to cling to hope. Instead I've been building our relationship, getting closer to her, so that when the time comes for us to talk about it we'll have the common ground.

"How do I work on the relationship? By being myself and not running away from the emotions in a situation. With this mother I remember when she told me that the neurologist had informed her that he thought her child had no chance of ever improving. We sat there together and cried. It was the only response that made any sense emotionally.

. . .

"I love the variety of cultures in this community. We have big Latino, Cambodian, and Gypsy communities. Most problems that parents come in with are socially related, and a lot of it is cultural. I mean, I have never had a Latino family come in with a question about toilet training. They just seem to handle it very well. But they often come in with sleep problems because they carry their babies all the time, and the baby never learns to settle down by herself.

"I'm pretty direct in how I talk to parents about these problems because I know that I have credibility. The credibility comes from the quality of care we provide the community. Everyone knows they are going to be treated with respect and get quality care here.

"So when a family comes in with a four-year-old who is really obese, and that's a pretty common issue, I let them explain what's going on. They'll say, 'He only eats McDonald's and other junk food.' Then I say, 'Is that so? You mean, he drives himself over to McDonald's?' They laugh, and they get the point.

"The most interesting people are always the ones who have had to overcome something in life. That may be why I'm impatient with people in my generation who are caught up in their own lives who complain about all the little things and just don't realize that they are actually very fortunate.

"Last week one of my patient's mothers surprised me by inviting me to her house for lunch. A lot of doctors wouldn't go. They would say it wasn't professional, or they didn't have time. But I really wanted to go. Her husband took off work. Her daughter was there. We had a very nice time. And I got so much pleasure out of doing it. This was a mother whose daughter had recurrent ear infections. Nothing serious, but we managed to get them under control. She was grateful and she wanted to express that to me. It meant a lot.

"That's what you get out of investing in your relationships with families. They let you into their lives, and you learn a lot about how to live your own. It's something that benefits me more than anyone. It keeps me from burning out. It keeps me from getting out of balance with my own life and my own problems. It is why I am in medicine in the first place and the key is not to forget it."

The Literary Doctor

❧

Clifton Cleaveland, M.D., 62, general practitioner,
Chattanooga, Tennessee

Eugene Arnold, Ph.D., 69, psychologist,
Chattanooga, Tennessee

❧

PATIENT

Eugene Arnold has been Dr. Cleaveland's patient for 29 years. In recent years he has been treated for a heart attack, cerebral hemorrhages, and pulmonary embolisms.

. . .

"It's friend-to-friend when I see Dr. Cleaveland He's a few years younger than me, but not much. I feel like he's a very good doctor, of course, but that he's also got the wisdom that comes with age. He fits here in Chattanooga and he fits with me. He's a gentleman and a gentle man. And he knows how to pass the time enjoyably, and that can be an art.

"As a matter of fact, I saw him today and the technician in his office drew some blood. He put a piece of cotton on my arm and the only thing he had to wrap around it was this big, pink-colored bandage. Cliff says, 'Well, Gene, I can see by the fact that you are willing to wear that, you don't have any doubts about your manhood.'

"I said that I didn't have any doubts, but I didn't know about everyone else.

" 'Then you better roll your sleeve down,' he said.

"That's the way it is with him. He has a relaxed, involved way of interacting. So when you talk, you talk about everything. If I say something about the former Romania or Bulgaria, he knows about it. If I say something in French, he'll answer me in French. Today we solved all of President Clinton's problems and still had time to talk about Africa.

"It's this way because he feels comfortable in what he's doing, and because he makes you feel comfortable too. He's direct. He tells you what's going on with your body, but he also offers hope. He says, 'This is what's going on, and here are your alternatives.' There is always hope.

"And you can tell him anything. There have been several

times since he's been my doctor that I thought I wasn't going to make it. Once he quoted the Twenty-third Psalm to me. He said, 'Now Gene, you've walked through the shadow of the valley of death several times and come out all right. You should be grateful.'

"It really wasn't what I wanted to hear at that moment. I told him. I said, 'If you will refrain from preaching, I will refrain from practicing medicine.' He agreed.

"When you know Dr. Cleaveland, you know that he's involved with you and your family, not just with what's wrong with you. I think he does feel a sort of love for his patients and he shows it. When I was sick, Cliff made a point of putting his hand on my son's shoulder and talking to him very kindly. My son is six-foot, five inches tall, but Cliff showed him concern as if he was his son.

"The fact that he goes to funerals is not surprising. Cliff doesn't try to avoid anything. I think he wants to be supportive of the family when one of his patients dies. But I also think he keeps himself aware of death—of all of life's realities—because it helps him to live a better life himself. He is aware of how precious life is, and he enjoys every minute. He's leaving for England soon, where's he's going on a 115-mile walking tour. He and his wife have been preparing for it for a while by walking in the mountains here. That's the way he is. He's really involved in all sorts of things.

"Lately he's been talking about his new granddaughter and how perfect everything about her is, her tiny fingers and tiny nails.

"Cliff is intelligent and he is scholarly. He stays very current in medicine. But he still is able to express something very simple about the beauty of a baby's hands. He has a gentleness and a way of focusing on you that lets you know that he is with you and no one else. He sees you as a person who has a body, yes, but also a soul and a spirit.

"Does it help get you better care? I think so. I know that when Cliff asks me a question I give him a much fuller, more detailed response than I would otherwise. I'm not afraid to open up, to tell him exactly what I'm feeling, emotionally or physically. That's what everyone's relationship with their doctor should be like. I'm glad I have it. In fact, the only worry I have with Cliff is that he might retire."

DOCTOR

Born in 1936, Clifton Cleaveland was raised in Columbia, South Carolina. As a boy he was enthralled by family legends about two great uncles who were both doctors. The Southern tradition of storytelling, and the art of active listening, which he learned as a child, are central to his relationships with patients. Every year he moderates a weekend retreat for doctors and writers in which the role of the story in medicine is explored.

On the day we met, Dr. Cleaveland invited us to join him in attending a funeral for one of his older patients. "I find myself going to a lot of these lately," he quipped. "It's not because of the way I practice medicine, but because of my age."

"I remember lazy Sundays, listening to people tell stories after dinner. They included as many long pauses as text, and I savored the process of revelation. You'd hear about the boll weevils and murders, about a great uncle who built a great fortune, and about a son who squandered it. It was the way to learn, and you learned everything.

"I saw this with my father. He was a traveling insurance salesman. He was extremely successful, mainly because he listened. His territory included all these small towns in West Georgia. He would call on someone and sit with them for a long time. He didn't make a sales pitch. He just had a conversation.

"Patients are no more generic than doctors. They are all different. They all have a story, which is just as important as any symptoms that are evident in an examination. You can't say, Mr. X has hypertension, period. You have to say, Mr. X has hypertension dot, dot, dot. That means you are waiting for the rest of the story, and the diagnosis isn't accurate until you get it. I want them to understand the importance of their stories too. That's why I tell people to keep journals. I even prescribe the reading of a specific novel, from time to time. Often it's Anne Tyler. Or Faulkner. It helps them understand themselves. One patient, a nurse who had cancer, left her journal to me when she died. I considered that a great honor.

"The story is not a product, but a process that is still unfolding. It's about family, sexual orientation, addictions, everything. And it's more than words. It's in how someone holds their body, how they look at you, how they respond to things in life. And sometimes it takes a long time. You don't get the story of a person by sitting down and taking a medical history. You have to establish a climate of trust. Then you receive the story gradually. Sometimes this happens very slowly.

"I remember a patient named Lena, who I treated for years.

Lena had already worn out several doctors. Her main problem was a terrible headache. We had frequent scheduled visits, but often the headaches would be so terrible that between these appointments she would just appear at the office because it hurt so much. I'd put her in a dark room with ice bags applied to her eyes or her head. A nurse would stay with her and basically talk her down. It could take hours, but we never stopped trying to make her suffering less. That's part of being a physician.

"Objectively, there were no real organic reasons for these headaches. But there was no question that they were real and they hurt very much. I remember that she would cry and say, 'Why is God doing this to me?'

"Lena was very withdrawn. Taking her history was like playing connect the dots. She'd offer a little bit and then withdraw. I was waiting for a breakthrough. One day she came in and she had cut off all her hair. This was shocking because she had had such long, beautiful hair. It turned out that she had a niece who was going through chemotherapy and she had lost all of her hair. This had moved Lena to take off hers.

"Lena then told me that she had survived the concentration camps in Nazi Germany, but her sister had not. One of her most important memories was at the end of the war, lying on the floor of a stable in Dachau with her hair frozen to the ground. She was losing consciousness and had a vision of God on a horse.

"Listening to this, I began to realize what might be going on. With the headaches, Lena had been putting herself in isolation. She had felt tremendous survivor guilt for making it through the war when so many people did not. The headaches were a way that she punished herself and put herself back in the camps. Seeing her niece without hair was a reminder of this.

Cutting her hair was another way of staying in the camps and not surviving when others had died.

"Her story was important because it really helped me understand what might be going on, symbolically. Lena agreed to see a psychiatrist and gradually these disabling headaches began to go away. I am sure they would have continued if I hadn't established a relationship with Lena that was strong enough for her to feel comfortable finally telling me her story.

"It's not just the doctor-patient relationship that matters. Within families you can see that relationships—especially between spouses—are also very powerful. If an older patient comes in and says his wife just died, I watch him pretty carefully. Recently a longtime patient's wife died of breast cancer. He had survived cancer himself fifteen years ago. She dies and then KABOOM, his cancer returns with mestasteses all over.

"I'm noticing this kind of thing happening more as my patients get older. Of course I am getting older too. It's sort of poetic, how we are passing through life together, my patients and me. Now I find that my role is to help them get through this stage of life, to manage it well. This doesn't just mean fixing things that go wrong. With aging that's not always easy. Often a patient's children will demand that I fix everything wrong with their eighty- or ninety-year-old parent. My job then becomes to explain to them that this is aging and it's not an easily reversed biological process.

"At this stage I also find I'm helping a fair number of patients die the way they want to. They make the decisions. If they don't want a breathing tube or other procedures to prolong life, they don't get them.

"Here again, the relationship makes all the difference. It's easier to go along with those wishes when you really know someone, and you can see that what they are choosing is consistent with the way they have lived the rest of their lives. At this time I'll often do house calls, because it puts me on the patient's territory. He feels most comfortable, can be himself and be in charge. I remember recently visiting a patient who was dying from prostate cancer. As I came in he was waving his hands to the music he was playing. He said he was conducting the music he had picked out for his funeral. 'This time I get to play what I like, and everyone has to listen,' he said.

"Going to funerals is important to me. I have to go, for closure for myself and sometimes because the spouse or others in the family are also my patients. I want to show them I care. This is probably the last bit I can say about the doctor-patient relationship.

"Doctors who avoid funerals, don't allow themselves to grieve always get in trouble because those feelings come out in anger or depression much later. You have to know and share your own feelings. The irony is that acknowledging the pain you feel yourself, as the doctor, is the only way to avoid much worse pain in the future. Getting involved, caring, is as good for the doctor as it is for the patient."

PART FIVE

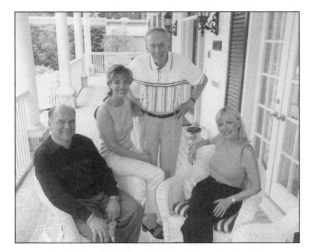

Dr. John Stehlin and Dr. Peter de Ipolyi

The
Friends

All His Children

❦

Arnold Gold, M.D., 73, pediatric neurologist,
New York, New York

Joey Trout, son of Marcia Lewis, 47,
a musician and teacher, New York, New York

❦

PATIENT

Joey Trout became Dr. Gold's patient in 1995. He was two and a
half years old. Twenty-one months later he died of the brain
tumor that Dr. Gold initially diagnosed. In that time he received

chemotherapy and radiation treatment, and he was treated at a controversial clinic where an unproven medicine is used to fight all types of cancers. He enjoyed a period of remission that carried him almost through the summer of 1996. A recurrence, which began in August, led to his death that November.

"The first thing that made all of our doctors, but especially Dr. Gold, special is that they really suffered with us. You could see it on their faces. They got attached to Joe and did everything they could for him. When he died, it hit them all pretty hard. They were wonderful as people first; then they were wonderful doctors.

"We first saw Dr. Gold on a snowy Saturday. Our pediatricians had already recommended we see him, because Joe had started to tilt his head off to one side when he was walking, and they knew he should see a neurologist. But when Saturday came and we noticed that one eye was dilated more than the other, they sent us immediately to the hospital. By the way, one of our pediatricians had had a cousin who was saved from a brain tumor by Dr. Gold, so we had even more reason to want him.

"On that day Dr. Gold was snowed in at his home, but he directed the tests from there. When he finally made it to the hospital he wasn't dressed as a doctor but in clothes for going to a concert. He missed the concert and a dinner he was supposed to go to, to be with us.

"Dr. Gold is kind of ageless. He's got this white hair, and yet he interacts very nicely with children. One of the first things I noticed was that he used a higher-pitched voice with children and he had great toys. Some doctors just use any old thing, but he had these Sesame Street finger puppets that were perfect, just what kids love. And as he was working with Joe, when he got stuck and couldn't get him to respond, he was able to let me help with it being no big deal. It was seamless. All of a sudden we were a team. It was a partnership from the very start.

"He was extremely nice, but he was also very direct. He told us there was a mass in his brain, but we needed more tests to tell us exactly what it was and what we could do. It was devastating. We had to stay there in the hospital and wait until Monday when we could find out everything. But Dr. Gold did one thing that helped very much. He gave us his home phone number. He said we could call him at any time of day, no matter what, and he would speak to us. We didn't use it that night, but just having it was a lifeline.

"After all the tests were done, when we finally talked about what was really going on, he said that the diagnosis was more final than others. Joe had the kind of tumor that couldn't be operated on and would probably not be cured by radiation or chemotherapy. There was a 99.9 percent chance that this tumor would kill him and, if it didn't, it would be because it had been diagnosed improperly.

"Then he said one thing that was very liberating for us in the long run. He probably didn't even recognize he was doing it. But he told us that we should go out and do as much research as possible and try everything we could try. 'You need to dot your i's and cross your t's so that you know in your hearts you did everything.' We took him seriously, and we got a lot of peace out of knowing we had done it.

"The other thing that he said we should do—and this we agreed with immediately—was that we should focus as much as possible on the quality of Joe's remaining life, not the quantity. There was a meeting of the minds there.

"There's one other thing about Dr. Gold giving us his phone number, and that's the sense of empowerment it gives you. Once, when Joe had had a very hard day in the hospital and I had finally gotten him to sleep, a group of residents and interns showed up to say they wanted to take him for a test. Now this test had been delayed all day. It was ten o'clock. He had just fallen asleep.

"I challenged them. I asked them if it was medically necessary that it be done right away. They gave me these bureaucratic answers about how they were supposed to do it, but they wouldn't say it was medically necessary. So I said that I had Dr. Gold's home number and I would call him right now. If he said it had to be done, then we would do it. If he didn't, we wouldn't.

"Well, they did not want me to call him at home. They backpedaled right away. They called the doctor who was in charge of their service and quickly came back to say that they could do the test tomorrow.

"Dr. Gold's reputation was one thing that helped us all the time. We were traveling once and Joe got sick in California. The doctor we saw knew of Dr. Gold and it made him take notice. In the hospital, whenever they saw that Joe was Dr. Gold's patient they were even nicer than they usually were. Once we were even in a stationery store and Joe was buying a card for Dr. Gold. A woman in line heard us talking about him and she interrupted and said, 'My son was treated by Dr. Gold. He's wonderful.'

"Joe got very attached to him. One day it seemed like every doctor in the hospital was coming in and poking and checking him. Joey got up and went into the hallway and started running for the exit. I ran after him, and when I caught him I said, 'Where do you think you're going?' He said, 'Find doctor. Big doctor with white hair.'

"Dr. Gold really did treat Joe like he was his own. When decisions were made, he thought about him that way. Not all doctors let themselves get this close. I remember when it came time for us to sign the do–not–resuscitate order, when Joe was dying. I asked one of the doctors what he would do if it were his child. He froze, with this stunned look on his face. He had obviously not thought like that before.

"With Dr. Gold it came naturally. He sometimes even referred to him as Joey Gold. This came up when Joe started chemotherapy. He did very poorly and got very sick. The doctors all had a big meeting, and Dr. Gold was very firmly against continuing. He didn't see that it was doing any good and it was making him so sick. He was also the one who advocated treating Joe with radiation.

"The radiation was controversial because they usually don't give it to someone under age three. It can damage them too much and really affect their intelligence. But Dr. Gold kept saying that where the tumor was located, there wouldn't be much to damage and that if they didn't try it, the tumor was going to kill him anyway, so what's to lose?

"The radiation oncologist was hesitant to do it at first, and the schedule to get the treatment was already filled up. Then Dr. Gold talked to her and it happened that afternoon. She did it for Dr. Gold, and you know what? It really worked for a while. That's when Joe started to improve a lot.

"When you are faced with something that's supposed to be a fatal illness, you are willing to try anything, and Dr. Gold said we could look at every option. He said that if we found something he would look at it and if it wasn't going to hurt, support us in trying it.

"We did get a lot of information about this controversial doctor in Texas. He read it all. He was pretty skeptical, but he said it wasn't going to hurt Joe. In fact, the main thing he was worried about was that we'd go broke paying the bills. We went ahead and it worked for a while, but then he got sick again.

"At the end, Dr. Gold was pretty clear about the fact that Joe was dying. I was prepared to take care of him at home and that's what we did. Dr. Gold came to a memorial concert we had after he died, and he has stayed in touch ever since. He calls just to see how we are doing. Sometimes I stop by his office after five o'clock, and I can see him for a few minutes.

"This may sound a little strange, but one of the hard things about this is not seeing so much of him and all the other wonderful people who helped us. Dr. Gold gave us the tools to go through this trial without regrets. He's a very wise man. He cared for our whole family, including Joe's older brother Mike. If you could invent a doctor to help you through something like this, you would invent Dr. Gold."

DOCTOR

The son of two lawyers, Arnold Gold was born in 1925 and raised to do "better than my best." After studying bacteriology at the University of Texas, he found it difficult to enroll in medical school in the U.S., in part because a limited number of Jewish students were accepted each year. Though he spoke no French, he accepted an offer to study in Switzerland and acquired the language in his first three months abroad. His residencies included obstetrics at a hospital in Dublin, Ireland, where he rode a bicycle to the homes where he delivered babies.

Back in the U.S., Dr. Gold was influenced by working at New Orleans Charity Hospital's polio ward under Dr. Margaret Smith. He practiced rural medicine in Hazard County, Kentucky, before settling into the nascent specialty of neurology at Columbia Presbyterian Hospital in New York.

"It is sometimes amazing to see how complicated cases can be and how the doctor's relationship with the patient—and the patient's illness—can affect the entire family. That's one thing you notice over the years. Everyone is connected, and the way that I handle a case has an effect that ripples out to touch many people. As a child neurologist you always have three patients really. The child and the two parents. Sometimes it's more, when there's an extended family involved.

"A good example of this is a mother who came in with a child—a boy one and a half years old—who showed some paralysis of the left side. She was really focused on a bruise he had on his head, which was caused by a fall he had had a while ago. The fall had taken place when the child was with a baby-sitter.

"Well, the mother's in-laws had been very hard on her for leaving the child with a baby-sitter even before this happened. I could see she was upset. 'They would like to see me barefoot and pregnant all the time,' she told me. Well, I knew it wasn't caused by this bump, but she was certain. We did an MRI that showed he had a tumor near the spinal cord. Even this did not convince her. It took a long time to convince her that it wasn't her fault. She didn't have to feel guilty. It was just one of those things that happen. As she began to trust me, to believe in our relationship, she eventually accepted it and let go of that guilt.

"In this specialty you often meet people in extreme circumstances. Their pediatrician has referred them because he is worried about something. They are feeling threatened and vulnerable. It's a very unusual relationship. You are a total stranger, but they are hoping that you will be very wise and very skilled.

"In this situation I try to build on three qualities: trust, respect, and 100 percent honesty. I don't have to write very detailed notes about what I did or didn't tell a patient because I know that I always tell everything I can as soon as I know it. There's never anything I have to worry about blurting out because I never hide anything.

"It has to be mutual. I offer those things to my patient and their parents, and I expect to get them in return. Usually this isn't that difficult to establish. After all, we're in a serious situation and we all want the same outcome. I make people understand that right away, that I really am on their side.

"It's all made more complicated by the fact that many cases start out with a seemingly minor problem, but when the cause is discovered to be something major, it hits people hard. I remember seeing this child who was about two or three. His name was Joey. He had been referred by a pediatrician who noticed he was blinking one eye more often than the other. At first they thought conjunctivitis, but it didn't clear up. That's scary. When I examined him I found one pupil was dilated, and his head was tilted. By the sound of the symptoms, it doesn't seem like it should be something bad, but it was. It was a tumor at the brain stem. Almost 100 percent of these patients die.

"We all began as total strangers, but in a very short time became very close. His mother was totally devoted. So was the father. The first thing I did was tell her that it was a privilege for me to see her and to treat her son. I told her right away that I would treat her child as if he were my own and that all my energy and experience would be devoted to him. His name, for me, became Joey Gold.

"We treated Joey first with radiation, which did work. The head tilt disappeared and he became bright and alert. We were all very happy with this, but I also knew from experience that this was probably not permanent. That's the honesty. I'm not in a popularity contest. I told his mother that usually it all comes back. It was hard for her to hear, but she's a very proactive person, and she immediately began researching all the other treatment modalities.

"When it came back I explained everything, including the chemotherapy and its side effects. Immediately there was this grief and pain. I said, 'You are not going to go through this alone. I will be with you every step. You can question me. You can scream at me. You can argue with me. And if you want to see someone else, I will help you.'

"This is not minor league stuff. These parents are giving me their children to make them well, but I haven't got much at my disposal to use. There's radiation, chemotherapy, and sometimes surgery. That's it. In the end what I also offer is support and guidance. I also meet with siblings and answer their questions. They want to know how to interact with their brother.

"Joey did die, at about age five. I attended the memorial service and I shared in the sorrow. But I didn't feel like a failure. I felt that I had made a substantial contribution to the life of that child and to his family. They felt that way too, and it helped me with my own grief. That's something I don't understand about the doctors who run away from these kinds of cases. They miss the opportunity to be a positive part of people's lives when they need it most. That is a gift.

"Joey's mother still comes by my office once in a while, just to talk. We talk about her other son and how she's raising him. I'm very grateful for our relationship. I treasure it.

"Usually it is the child who has the most severe problem that draws us closest. Maybe it is the sense of emergency, of an extreme danger, that brings people so close together. And often it lasts forever. I had a Mennonite family come down from Canada to have me treat a child who turned out to have a malignant tumor. This was way back, before the CAT scan. The child died, but the family continues to visit me every year.

"Another family brought me an eight-year-old with a spinal cord tumor. This child made it. The father, who turned out to be quite wealthy, showed up at my office one Christmas with a check that he put on my desk. 'I'd like you to do something for children,' he said. It was for ten thousand dollars.

"At the time I had been talking a lot about the fact that the human side of medicine, the emphasis on patients and doctors relating compassionately was dying. We were making great technological advances: new medicine, new machines, new procedures. But we were losing touch with how to ease suffering, how to connect.

"When this check arrived, my wife said it was time for me to either do something or shut up. We used it to start a foundation to promote the humane practice of medicine. Every year the same father brings another check. They've gotten bigger. And we use the foundation to go to medical schools and encourage them to train young doctors to be compassionate and not hide behind technology. They were getting so involved with CAT scans and MRIs that they were forgetting the people.

"One of my messages is that in these relationships with patients we get all of the unexpected, exciting things that make life enjoyable. Every interaction we have with a patient or family is an opportunity for an adventure. So many things happen because we open ourselves up to others. That's how I went to Europe, how I learned I liked to work with children, how I found the specialty of neurology. Every relationship you begin is an opportunity for something exciting and rewarding. I don't turn away, even when I know it may be painful later on. There's too much for me and the patient and their family to gain."

"Don't Just Do Something, Sit There"

⤺

Jamie Van Roen, M.D., 46, oncologist
and AIDS-treatment specialist, Chicago, Illinois

Dan Thomas, 39, cabinetmaker and artist,
Chicago, Illinois

⤺

PATIENT

Dan Thomas probably learned to be a patient while he watched his mother cope with Krohn's disease, a chronic inflammatory disease of the intestines. Born in 1959, Thomas was six years old when his mother was given the diagnosis. Refusing to accept that there was nothing to be done, she altered her diet, even grew her own vegetables, as part of her own care. She fared much better than her doctors predicted, and set an example for assertiveness and hopefulness that her son would follow years later when he was diagnosed with AIDS.

"I introduce Jamie as the person who helped save my life. She likes to say that I did it all, but I know that it's not true. We did it together. One of the most important things Jamie did was give me hope, along with the facts. A person with AIDS has to know that there's a strong possibility of living.

"Jamie was the person who told me I had lymphoma. My partner Tom had just died, and I was absolutely flattened by fatigue. I had put off getting an AIDS test because my insurance was not stable. My other doctor had been giving me vitamin B shots to keep me going, but I was still so exhausted that I couldn't even make it up the stairs. I was referred to Jamie, and she said she'd have to see if I had lymphoma. After the test, she was the one who gave me the news. With that, it was official that I had AIDS.

"She was very good in the way she handled it. She talked about what we were going to do to fight the lymphoma, but she was also willing to listen to me talk. A lot of the time I needed to talk about Tom. It may have seemed like it had nothing to do with my medical care, but it had a lot to do with how I was feeling. That's the thing about Jamie. She doesn't just ask about your symptoms. She asks about your feelings and then she listens, because she actually cares.

"But Jamie also reveals things about herself. I heard a little about her husband and her children. She also once told me something very touching. She said that she had never realized that two people of the same sex could love each other as deeply as Tom and I had. I knew she was telling me that to show that her attitudes were changing. She was willing to admit that she had had a preconceived idea about gay people and it was changing. I respected her for that and I took what she said as a compliment.

"We also talked a lot about how far we would go with treatment. A lot of doctors don't know when to stop. Tom's doctor had tried everything to keep him going. He was on a ventilator for three months. The doctor just wouldn't let him go. It was terrible. Jamie believes in fighting, in fighting hard, but she doesn't try to deny that death can happen. She doesn't like it, but she accepts it as part of life. A lot of doctors don't, and I think their patients feel like they are letting them down if they get sicker.

"When my lymphoma came back, I was really upset. I think it affected Jamie too. She hugged me every time I saw her, and no matter how many people were in her waiting room, she would focus only on me and never rush through an appointment.

"During the second round of chemo I got very discouraged. I was having a very hard time. At that point she gave me her home phone number and said I should use it if I had to. I did, twice. It was when I was really sick and I didn't know if I could go on. She was very positive with me. She told me I had come a long way and that there wasn't too much more to go. She made me want to be the poster boy for surviving with AIDS. I think it helped a lot.

"Jamie's attitude also rubbed off on the hospital staff. It got so that the hospital was a safe haven for me. I think that's the way it's supposed to be. She would come in in the morning and we would talk about everything. She'd give me a hug before she left. I think she never forgot that I was a person underneath all the problems. She treated me like a person, not like a disease.

"When you have a life-threatening illness, you want someone who is very good at what they do, but can also function as a close partner. I mean, in that kind of crisis people get very close. Jamie has a way of doing that perfectly. Her medical expertise and our relationship saw me through two bouts of chemotherapy and many pneumonias. Now I've been stable for more than a year and I'm living evidence that you can live with AIDS. I've done it all with the help of Jamie. She's a tough little cookie, but a sweet one too."

DOCTOR

Born in 1952 and raised in the city of Chicago, Jamie Van Roen worked as a union telephone operator as a high school student. She interrupted her college education for a year of travel and study: French cooking in London and radical politics with Ivan Illich in Mexico. This life experience is one of two main influences that have determined her approach to the doctor-patient relationship. The other is her extensive work with terminally ill patients.

A small, thin woman with boyishly short and graying hair, Van Roen was interviewed on the eve of her departure for Geneva and the annual international conference on AIDS. Her office at Northwestern University Hospital was decorated with family photos and a little glass bull—a symbol of her tenacity—that was a gift from a patient.

"In college I studied special education and I helped to run a summer camp for disturbed children. That work was with a psychiatrist who was on the faculty. I loved the work, but in a way it wasn't big enough. I wanted more of a challenge, intellectually and academically, but I also valued human relationships. Medicine and oncology was the perfect fit. The science is exciting and ever-changing. But the doctor-patient relationship also means something. You don't cure people by addressing emotional issues, but you do make people feel better, make their lives better, if you treat the whole person.

"In oncology patients have to make choices, and often they are choices about how they will die. I talk about that very early in our relationship because I know that when the time comes, they will have thought about it more. Most patients say that we should do everything that provides them with a reasonable quality of life. I tell them very specifically what intubation is, and what dying on a ventilator can be like. You can't talk, and you can't eat. And I ask them to identify someone who will make the decisions they want made when the time comes.

"At the beginning most people say they don't want much done if they can't have a high quality of life. But quality of life at the beginning of their illness may mean being active, while quality of life at the end may be just being able to communicate. I want to have an open relationship so they can tell me that their thinking has changed. So they can tell me what they want.

"There's an old adage in the hospice movement: Don't just

do something, sit there. That's how you establish a relationship. You sit with a person and you listen. You don't rush them out of your office. You listen to even the smallest things. And then, over time, they open up more and more. Everyone is more comfortable opening up to a friend rather than a stranger. I'm their doctor, but I'm a friend too. I care.

"These relationships are real. And there is one case where we got so close that I couldn't treat someone. Dan came in to see me with lymphoma. I saw him through treatment. He went into retirement, like a lot of people with AIDS who I've seen. Anyway, we got pretty close. He and a lot of my patients knew that I was about to adopt a baby. On the day that I went to pick up the child, the mother changed her mind. She backed out. I was devastated. Well, a lot of my gay patients sent me flowers when they found out.

"The first thing I do to try to make the relationship real is teach them to complain. I tell them that I don't know what it's like to be the patient, to have cancer. It's a matter of control. Patients often feel like they have lost control of everything. I try to give it back.

"Sometimes it's a small thing that matters to someone. I was with a guy recently who was into his first cycle of chemotherapy. He was hesitating before I examined him. I could see it. So we talked about it. I told him I would let him decide about taking his clothes off. He chose to do it, but it was his decision. That may seem like a small thing, but it wasn't for him.

"There are big things, too. One patient comes to mind. I had seen him for years and we knew each other pretty well. We ran in similar circles. I saw him a lot at my favorite restaurant.

"Anyway, he was the first one who asked me to help him commit suicide. We talked about it over several months. I remember visiting him at his house once. He was in the garden. He was blind from his CMV [a viral infection associated with AIDS], but he still enjoyed the garden, the sun on his face, hearing the birds. He never did choose suicide, and I wouldn't have helped him if he did. But he knew I wouldn't condemn him for considering it. I mean, I knew he could do it himself. You can find out about it in books. I wasn't telling him he couldn't make that choice. I respected his right to do what he wanted. In the end, it seemed like what he really needed most was the conversation we had about it—open and honest—over a long period of time.

"AIDS taught me about the importance of being willing to touch patients. Most of my patients have been from the gay community. There's a lot of openness to feelings, a lot of touching. And there's a real direct effort to deal with death on an individual basis. You learn to accept death as natural for everyone, and you accept that. Our lives are stories, really. Relationships and stories. All stories have endings. When someone dies peacefully, the way they want to because they were able to orchestrate it, that's a happy ending.

"Learning to look at my patients' deaths this way is how I avoid burning out. You can't help people who are dying if you haven't resolved your own issues with death in your own mind.

"I go to the homes of my patients when they are dying. Usually patients and their friends and families want to show me that this person is more than the disease, that they have an entire life. People want to show me who they are and who they were. And they want to die in the same way they lived.

"I remember one patient who said to me when he was doing pretty well that he wanted to die alone. Many months later he was in a hospice. I went to see him and we talked for a while. A lot of his friends were there. At some point he told us all to leave, go out for dinner. We all said good-bye, and while we were out he died, just like that. People have more control than you think.

"When people don't have control it can be pretty horrible. I lost my father a year and a half ago. We were very close. When I was young he was the one I could talk to about anything, sex, anything, and even as an adult I spoke to him every day. He had gone into the hospital after a heart attack. He wanted to go ahead with a procedure, a catheterization. He wanted to try anything. The cardiologist called me and said, 'I'm more likely to kill him than help him, and if I don't, he's not likely to get any better.'

"Now in a case like that I would be very honest with a patient. I'd say, 'There's really no way we're going to help you with another catheterization.' But the cardiologist didn't tell my father that. So my father went through it. He spent the whole day hooked up to all this technology, and then he died in the catheterization lab. His whole last day was spent doing that instead of being with the people he loved.

"In a way, the situation was caused by the doctor. A lot of doctors get focused on the disease and forget the person. Then, whenever one of their patients dies it's a crisis, because they are not prepared to deal with the people.

"It's about doctors taking care of people all the way through. You have to be honest and listen when they talk to you. I've heard colleagues say that when they are rushed they don't ask patients if anything is bothering them, because they feel like they are running behind. But if you listen to patients from the beginning, establish that trust, you won't get overwhelmed by your patients later on. In fact, they don't call on you as much, they actually call on you less. They call less because they are confident that you will be there when they really need you.

"People tell you everything, and they make very specific choices. When I work with them and they finally die, I can walk away saying I gave them everything I could in that relationship. That's how you avoid burning out.

"It doesn't always work out. I make mistakes. One patient in particular comes to mind. It was a woman who was in hospice. She became comatose, but I knew it was possible to wake her up by simply treating her with fluids and calcium. The way I presented it to her husband he had no choice. He had to approve of it.

"Looking back, I realized that I really wasn't sure that was what she wanted. I realized that in part, I woke her up because I wanted to say good-bye. And you know, when she did wake up, one of the first things she said was, 'What did you do that for?'

"I've learned so much working with people with AIDS because it is such a sensitive subject. I realized that when I noticed there were times when I didn't want to risk saying that I was a doctor when I called for someone. That's when I found out that just saying I was Jamie, rather than 'doctor' was a good idea. The 'doctor' can also be a barrier to people. I only use it now when I want a reservation at a restaurant."

Well-Trained Friends

෴

John Stehlin, M.D., 75, and Peter de Ipolyi, M.D., 53,
cancer surgeons, Houston, Texas

Lin Mills, 49, interior designer, and Mary Epperson, 27, artist,
Houston, Texas

෴

LIN MILLS, PATIENT

Lin Mills was treated at the Stehlin Clinic for breast cancer. She
underwent a single mastectomy and reconstructive surgery. Her
primary doctor at the clinic is John Stehlin.

.   .   .

"My cancer was discovered in a routine mammogram. My doctor sent me to the oncologist that he thought was best. I remember when I went in there I was hoping for the best. The doctor said that the only possible treatment was a radical mastectomy, and no reconstructive surgery would be possible.

"I was in a state of shock, vulnerable, and upset. I had a lot of questions, but he didn't seem to want to answer them fully. He kept pressing me to make decisions about treatment before I felt like I had all the information.

"I left that doctor and went to five others, looking for someone who I could communicate with. They all offered sympathy but did nothing to assuage my fear. Instead they focused on the cancer and killing it. I left their offices feeling more afraid. I kept thinking about this friend of mine who wound up having a double mastectomy, and when it was all over her doctor was offended by her lack of gratitude.

"I waited a long time, at least an hour, past my appointment time the first time I saw Dr. Stehlin. But I didn't know that during that time he was looking at my charts, meeting with a radiologist and a surgeon and going over everything. When we met, the first thing he said was, 'Sweetheart, I'm not worried about you. You are going to live a long life.'

"All of a sudden I realized that I had become clinically detached from what was happening to me and how serious it all was. He invited a whole team of people—I think there were seven of us—to go over my records for an hour. I suggested the idea of reconstruction, and he said, 'I think that's a wonderful idea.'

"The whole approach made me feel like I was part of a big team that was going to do everything possible for me. But they also treated me like I was a client, a valued person, and that I had the ultimate authority in every decision. It made me feel wonderful. Dr. Cohen, my surgeon, pledged to me that he would do his very best work.

"Immediately before my surgery Dr. Stehlin came to see me. I had told him that I didn't want Valium before the surgery because I wanted a clear mind. I said I would use meditation to relax instead. When he came in he gave me a big hug and said how proud he was of me and my relaxed heart rate. Then when I got into the operating room I looked around and saw all these faces of familiar people. They were the people I had picked to be there. It was like they were friends there to help me, and they did."

MARY EPPERSON, PATIENT

Mary Epperson's primary doctor at the clinic is Peter de Ipolyi.

Stricken by breast cancer in her mid-twenties, she was determined to learn every option available to her. She sought and found a doctor who would help her obtain a full cure that also left her body and her life as whole as possible.

"I had just gone through a change in insurance companies when I discovered the lump myself. I had to rush over to see a doctor I had never met before. I wanted to know if it was cancer and if it was, what we were going to do. He just took out this list and began going through the names of oncologists. He gave me the name of a doctor, but when I called they said I would have to wait six weeks for an appointment.

"I had worked as a massage therapist before, and I had some clients who had been through breast cancer. I did not want to wait and wonder for weeks about what was going to happen to me. I'm not that kind of person. I read up on things, I'm very interested in medicine. I take action.

"I had heard about Dr. Stehlin and Dr. de Ipolyi so I made an appointment. But when I got there, my insurance company hadn't yet approved payment. So I got on the phone with them right there. I could see Dr. D. waiting in the hallway for me. I could hear him tell the staff, 'Just send her back here. I want to see her. I don't care about the insurance. We'll work that out later. Send her back.'

"That impressed me. But what impressed me even more was that he and I immediately began working together on this. I said I wanted a needle biopsy. He said, 'When do you want it?' I said I wanted it right away, and he said he would schedule it for that afternoon. That told me that he knew what I was going through. He understood and he cared.

"Hearing him say that he didn't care about the insurance and that he just wanted to see me was very important, but something happened as I was leaving the appointment that made an even bigger impression. He followed me out and into the hallway, and we stopped for a minute to talk about how to handle the insurance problem. I leaned back against the wall with my hands behind my back and put a foot up behind me, against the wall. He leaned against the wall the same way, even putting the same foot up and putting his hands behind his back too.

"What he did was unconscious. It's called mirroring. And it shows someone has real empathy for you. I've read that 85 percent of communication is body language and I believe it. By his body language he was letting me know that he saw me completely as a person. He was interested in me as a person, not just a disease."

DOCTOR

John Stehlin authored one of the first articles on psychology and cancer care ever published in a major medical journal. In the thirty years since, Stehlin has continued to explore the doctor-patient relationship. He has paid close attention to the doctor side of the equation, focusing on the effect that a physician's expectations and motivations have on patients. Stehlin says an unusual opportunity—a grant that funded psychotherapy for him when he was a young doctor—began his lifelong interest in the psychology of medicine. Thin and a bit stooped with age, Stehlin speaks slowly, choosing his words with care.

Once a protégé of Dr. Stehlin, Peter de Ipolyi, M.D., is now his partner in a busy oncology practice and research center affiliated with St. Joseph's Medical Center in downtown Houston. Dr. de Ipolyi helped pioneer several cancer treatments. His surgical training included work with Houston heart surgeons Michael DeBakey and Denton Cooley. Tall and muscular, de Ipolyi communicates his energy and enthusiasm through a broad, beaming smile.

. . .

Stehlin

"I think it's very important to recognize that doctors expect certain rewards, satisfactions, from their relationships with patients. You want an emotional reimbursement. That's not bad. It's just real, a part of the relationship that should be recognized.

"Probably the best speciality for this is obstetrics. You get to build a close relationship with your patients over six to nine months. Then on the night that the baby is born you rush to the hospital, and then you can say to the mother, 'Here's your baby!' It's wonderful.

"In oncology you pour all of your time and energy—emotional and physical—into curing your patients. When you finish the operation you feel so good. The patient goes home thinking I'm God almighty. That feeling remains until she gets a recurrence. Then I'm negated. My omnipotence fails. Now what do I do? I realized that what I have to do is set different goals. Be something different than the omnipotent surgeon.

"What I am, really, is a trained friend for my patients. I'm someone who is going to help see them through this time. That's a very important thing. It means building a true relationship so the patient knows you as a person. I tell them right away that I don't have any magic. I am human, just like you. I make mistakes, too. But I do care about you. When a beautiful young person comes in and you discover the cancer and you know what their chances are, they have to know that you are pained too. Don't be afraid to show them your pain, because you care about them."

·   ·   ·

de Ipolyi

"This is something John and I talk about a great deal—The Trained Friend. I first heard about it twenty-five years ago. John told patients then that he couldn't treat them alone. The patient has to be a partner. He has to carry his load. The patient is not an object of the treatment, she is a participant. When a new patient comes in we formally welcome them to our team. The team is dedicated to your care, but you are an important part of the team and we make sure they know it."

Stehlin

"Doctors have to understand that they will have a tendency to turn patients into objects, especially if things are not going so well. I have done this myself. I'll have ten patients in the hospital that I am going to see on rounds. Those that you know are doing well you can hardly wait to see. Those who are not, you put off. I once went to see my patients and then went to have a sandwich, and in the middle of eating realized that I had forgotten to see one of them. Of course she was the one who was not doing so well. I had converted her into an object, a problem, and subconsciously just decided to forget her.

"To fight against this I try to make sure that I really know patients as people. I insist on it. If I can't establish that with someone, I really can't work with them. I remember this one patient, Michael, who flew in from Sacramento to see me. He always came with his wife. But he was one of those patients who seemed down all the time. He would come in and be all slumped over, very unresponsive, very uninvolved. He wouldn't even look me in the eye. I said, 'I can't relate to you Michael, if you don't look at me. You have to be alive. You have to carry on.'

"Michael decided to go to another doctor, and that's alright. But in other cases that approach has really worked. There was this one woman, Peggy, who was in the hospital and doing quite poorly. Usually she was very upbeat. She had a wig, because her hair had all fallen out, and she always dressed in a nice night gown and wore her makeup.

"Anyway, one day I went in and she had had a bad night. She was very disheveled. No makeup. Her hair piece was half on. She wasn't dressed nicely. She looked like she didn't care. Well, I told her, 'I can't work with this crap. Look at you. I won't have you giving up.' And I walked out.

"A little while later the nurses came to me and said, 'Peggy wants to see you.' I went back in and she was changed. Her hair piece was on straight, she had her makeup on and she had changed her clothes. She looked me right in the eye and said, 'Fuck you, John Stehlin.' I stepped back and applauded her."

de Ipolyi

"John is talking about being honest, as a person, in your relationship with a patient. It means sharing how you feel about something, along with the facts. Of course, how you share the facts is important, too. Patients must be told the truth, but you have to consider the tempo at which you deliver the truth.

"For example, after surgery a lot of patients don't even ask what you took out of them. It may seem strange, but it happens fairly often. In those cases you slow down. You give them the information as they ask for it. They will ask.

"The most important thing is to not hide behind the medicine and technology. I saw a patient here this morning who had had a questionable mammogram. I had treated her sister for breast cancer ten years ago. Now she had it. I had to go in and tell her we got a bad report back on her tests. She started crying and I have to say I started crying too. She's only thirty-six years old. She shouldn't have to deal with that. It's awful, and I just had a human response to it. It's not a problem. In fact, I find patients respect an honest reaction to their situation."

Stehlin

"It's important to understand that nothing creates more anger, for the doctor and the patient, than cancer. This is why solid tumor chemotherapists probably are the worst at relating to their patients. Their job is so frustrating; there are so many recurrences, and they often keep their feelings of anger and frustration inside. They are mad as hell, and they don't know what to do with their feelings. It costs a doctor a lot, emotionally, to do this kind of work. You can't do it at all if you don't recognize that."

How's Everything at Home?

❧

Roger Pelli, D.O., 50, family practitioner,
Presque Isle, Maine

Sybil Higgs, 74, homemaker, Presque Isle, Maine

❧

PATIENT

A homebound woman who receives few visitors, Sybil Higgs puts on her Sunday best and a full face of makeup for Dr. Pelli's visits, which are a blend of medical consultation and social therapy. Her main medical problem is chronic pulmonary obstruction, which was diagnosed following a heart attack in 1989. Asthmatic, she has been on oxygen therapy ever since.

"I've got so many problems. I've got a sister dying with cancer and I can't go see her. I got a daughter who's sick, and sometimes I call to talk to her and she doesn't want to talk to me.

"I guess there are people who care, though, like Dr. Pelli. Excuse my French, but he's the one doctor who I know gives a shit. He's not too busy for an old lady.

"Dr. Pelli has kept me going pretty good for an old lady. I've got chronic bronchitis, and I've had pneumonia several times. But he always takes care of me. He comes to see me and he calls me on the phone to check up afterwards.

"The most important thing about Dr. Pelli is that you never have to remind him about your problems. He knows me as a person, not a number. And he also knows that I'd prefer not to go into the hospital. They will foul up my medicine. I can take care of myself better at home, and if he can, he'll help me do it that way. Like the last time I had pneumonia. He gave me medicine, checked on me, and when he found it wasn't working gave me something else. It all worked out fine, because he listens.

"You always feel like you are getting his full attention, 103 percent. But he doesn't just focus on what's wrong with you. He'll talk, tell me about his children. I tell him about what's going on with me. It's not about making money or just getting through with the visit. In fact, he's told me that no matter what, as long as I'm alive, he'll take care of me, whether I can pay or not.

"I know I can count on Dr. Pelli to the end. I've made out a living will that says I don't want them to use anything extra to keep me alive. I'm a practical person. I believe when it's your time, it's your time. I don't want to waste a whole lot of money, and time—my time—attached to all those machines with my eyes closed. Dr. Pelli won't let that happen to me. I can count on him. He's a hell of a good guy."

DOCTOR

After graduating from a physician's assistant program at Dartmouth, Roger Pelli spent nearly a decade treating patients in an isolated corner of rural Maine. When physicians at the local hospital urged Pelli to attend medical school, the towns he served agreed to pay his tuition through their municipal budgets. With their backing, he graduated second in his class and returned to the north country town of Ashland, a family practitioner and the only doctor serving six communities strung along the Canadian border.

Today Roger Pelli is so well known in the community that during his one-day-a-week stint in the emergency room of the local hospital, he sees a full third of the unit's weekly patient load. He is so frequently interviewed by reporters for the one local TV station that they gave him a jacket embroidered with the station's logo and his name.

"You make a choice when you are a doctor. You decide whether you are going to really listen, get to know the patient, pay attention to the mental health component, or not. I began to learn this in the physician's assistant school. It was clear that some of the doctors were very distant, like they were apart. The doctor was king. Nurses stood up when they entered the room and gave them their chairs. I wanted none of that.

"The first history I ever took lasted four hours. Eventually I got past that. But I never stopped listening very carefully. My patients know that what's going on in their lives makes a difference to me. I always ask them the key question, 'How is everything at home?'

"They might not tell you something the first time, but if you always show an interest, they will start to trust. Then they might tell you something that has real medical significance. One example of this involved a woman patient of mine who was in her sixties. I had been trying to help her lose weight for a long time. She was married to this guy who was smaller than her, but very rough. Eventually she told me that he was threatening her. She was afraid that if she lost weight she wouldn't be able to defend herself. She was a devoutly Catholic woman, so divorce was out of the question. She planned on outliving him. I stopped focusing so much on her weight.

"You have to be aware of the context of your patient's life. People up here aren't as likely to have the same kind of stress and workaholism that people in cities have. I had this in mind when I treated an older man whose wife said he was fine, except he could no longer add up his gin-rummy hands.

"If he had lived someplace else, I might have thought it was stress. But he's one of those Mainers who is so relaxed you worry that if their house catches fire they won't get out in time. So I took it very seriously. We did all the tests. It turned out he had a brain tumor.

"Doctors are supposed to deal in the hard stuff, the worst things. When people really trust you they tell you the worst of what's happening, even if they are afraid or ashamed. It's what you hope your patients will be able to do, so you can help them.

"This happened once when a family called me to see an older man, severely alcoholic, who was living in an outhouse in the back of their property. It was a four-holer. He had put boards over the holes and made a place to lie down. There were nails in the wall all around it that he hung things on. He had a pot belly stove and three cats in there with him.

"Anyway, the family called and I went in to see him. He had pneumonia. He was so weak he had let the stove go out. In between the blankets were ice crystals. We got him over the pneumonia, but not the drinking. That's something you just have to accept, I guess. I used to see him walking into town for a bottle. He died at age eighty.

"Sometimes you can do a little more. I once saw a woman who complained of a lot of headaches and stomach pain. I found nothing. When I asked her what was going on at home she said she had had an affair. She was very upset. She said her husband was an alcoholic and they had a lot of problems. I tried to understand her. I think talking about it helped.

"A while after that I got a call from the same woman's mother-in-law. She said I had to come see her son, because he wasn't doing that well. That's all she said. I went to the house and he was there holding a shotgun. He was going to kill his wife, or himself. They had called me because they knew if they called the police that he would either get shot or go to jail. We talked for a long time. I told him that nothing would get better if he used the gun. Eventually he agreed. He was admitted to the psych ward at the hospital in Presque Isle. As far as I know, they are still together."

"Despite everything I'm saying, you have to realize that I really like my patients. If I showed up at someone's house on a snow-stormy night, most of them would insist I stay there. My practice has evolved into a population of patients that are like that.

"Doctors are still caregivers, not just healthcare-givers, but caregivers. That means being a real person in your patients' lives. It's much more rewarding for me, and I think it means better medical practice too."

Additional Resources on the Patient-Physician Relationship

BOOKS:

In the Country of Illness: Comfort and Advice for the Journey
by Robert Lipsyte
The Youngest Science: Notes of a Medicine-Watcher
by Lewis Thomas
Encounters Between Patients and Doctors: An Anthology
edited by John D. Stoeckle, M.D.
Anatomy of an Illness as Perceived by the Patient: Reflections on Healing and Regeneration
by Norman Cousins
Positive Doctors in America
by Mike Magee, M.D.

RECOMMENDED WEB SITES:

http://www.medscape.com/
http://www.pharminfo.com
http://www.mayohealth.org
http://www.healthlinks.net/bin/directory/index.cgi
http://www.sixsenses.com/
http://www.healthfinder.gov
http://www.nih.gov
http://www.os.dhhs.gov/
http://www.healthgate.com
http://www.guideline.gov
http://www.jama.com
http://www.nejm.org/content/index.asp
http://nhic-nt. health.org
http://www.personalMD.com
http://www.pfizer.com
http://www.positiveprofiles.com
http://www.cmwf.org/health_care/physrvy.html
http://www.ama.com
http://www.healthfinder.gov
http://www.healthweb.org
http://www.koop.com